Dedicated to William John Wieriman

In good times and in bad

He always loved his children

Table of Contents

Preface

Many books have been written about alcoholism and drug abuse. If this is your first book on addiction you will probably find it a bit dull. There are no personal stories on the tragedy of drug use or of persons who were redeemed. There is no long chapter on the use of drugs throughout the ages and how people's attitudes about drug use have fluctuated. There is nothing on how to convince someone to enter treatment or on detoxification. There is no detailed explanation of how the brain responds to opiates or how opiate agonists and antagonists work (medication-assisted treatment).

On the other hand, if you have read one or more books on addiction, you will probably be astounded. You will learn:

(1) That, to the best of my knowledge, there is no data to show that we are any better at preventing drug abuse or treating it now than forty years ago.
(2) Convincing people that drug abuse is a medical illness creates more problems than it solves.
(3) The much touted "Medication-Assisted Treatment" was available in the 1970's and Motivational Interviewing has a lot in common with Non-Directive Counseling done in the 1940's.
(4) The value of "evidence-based strategies" is minimal at best.
(5) Much of the addiction research is flawed.
(6) Cultural changes far exceed the impact of prevention and treatment.

(7) Once the half-a-billion dollars on the opioid crisis (2018) is spent, we will be back to square one.

Baring a major breakthrough, the only way to improve both prevention and treatment is the tried and true method of creating a system of feedback. State governments need to do referrals and follow-up, not treatment. My contribution to addiction research is represented by my proposed control groups. Without appropriate control groups, you cannot accurately measure what works. Furthermore, when any one study shows promising results, that study needs to be verified by a qualified statistician/researcher as to methodology and to other possible conclusions. If the study appears to be sound, it needs to be duplicated exactly by an uninterested party. No one wants to repeat someone else's study; that is why the federal government needs to pay for this.

I believe that the largest potential for gains in the treatment of substance abuse, excluding lawyers and politicians, are in the hands of the following entities in the order given:

1) State governments
2) Federal government
3) Public initiated actions
4) Treatment centers
5) Individuals involved in research
6) Former addicts
7) Others

My search of library books on substance abuse shows that the majority of books are written by those with the least potential impact. Unfortunately, I fall in the very last category. My only hope is that someone in one of higher categories will take notice of what I propose and follow through with action.

Introduction

Addictions to drugs and alcohol is nothing new. Nearly all historical periods and nearly all societies have had this problem. What is new, however, is that treating chemical addictions is a 35-billion-dollar business. The 21st Century Cures Act allows the United States government to spend 4.6 billion dollars in 2018 on the opioid crisis and an equal amount the next year (*Associated Press*, March 2018). Florida, the once opioid capital of the United States, received 27 million dollars and Louisiana, where I live, received 24 million dollars from the federal government. Neither Republicans or Democrats seem to object to spending money on a problem with little solid data on the effectiveness of treatment or prevention.

With all of this money being spent, you would think we knew what we were doing to solve this problem. Several books have recently come out on addiction. "*Overcoming Opioid Addiction*" (2018) by Adam Bisaga sees addiction as a medical problem while "*Unbroken Brain*" (2016) by Maia Szalavits claims addiction is learned. Other books such as "*The Addiction Solution*" (2018) by Lloyd Selern and "*Clean*" (2013) by David Sheff present a wealth of information but little new material in my opinion. *American Overdose* (2018) by Chris McGreal presents the recent pharmaceutical's political and legal history regarding opioids, especially OxyContin. *American Fix* (2018) by Ryan Hampton, is a plea for humane treatment and political action. *The Addiction Spectrum* (2018) by Paul Thomas and Jennifer Margulis promotes a wholistic approach to addiction treatment. They see proper nutrition, exercise, sleep and social interaction at least as helpful as medical treatment. *Never Enough* (2019) by Judith Grisel talks about how our brains process various drugs.

I do not claim to have a solution. Perhaps, some amazing breakthrough will come with the use of psychedelic drugs or some type of medical approach such as a vaccine. Scripps Research is presently working on a vaccine that get immune system antibodies to bind to heroin molecules thereby blocking the drug from reaching the brain.

The only thing I believe we can count on for improving the treatment of addiction is using the tried and true method of feedback. This feedback needs to be gathered by the states, not academia, from treatment centers. Academia has led federal and state administrators of addiction monies to believe in "evidence-based" programs. I will present several reasons why this only perpetuates a system that produces minimal gains.

Having worked for the federal government for years, I attended many seminars on management. The best one I ever attended was presented by physicist Dr. W. Edwards Deming. Dr. Deming helped turn Japan into an industrialized nation with a method called "Statistical Process Control" (SPC). SPC gathers data to see if a process is in or out of control. SPC would never set a goal of reducing accidents by 10%. SPC sets a goal of zero accidents with minimum variation. The goal of addiction treatment is zero relapse within a year with minimum variation. The fact that this goal may be unattainable in the near future (or ever) does not alter it.

Dr. Deming made me question the entire psychological practice of changing people. He believed in changing systems that in turn promote desirable behaviors. For example, if you want to reduce automobile accidents, you improve the safety of automobiles. Cameras reduce the number of speeders on the road, not lectures on good behavior. The simplest way to fight obesity would be a national tax on soft drinks. Want to reduce crime? Get rid of cash. It is hard to deal with illegal drugs with credit cards. We need to seriously consider cultural solutions to make a lasting impact on addiction rates; not just more money for school prevention programs and treatment facilities.

There are over twenty journals on addiction. I do not claim to be an expert on addiction. However, I do claim to understand statistics. I spent most of my life as a statistician including having taught a class at the University of Texas in San Antonio. Consequently, I will be presenting suggestions that will probably be new to you. Fortunately, you will not need a background in statistics to understand these.

A systems approach means more than using a variety of methods and services to treat addiction. It implies an integrated system of the following three services:

(1) Assessment and diagnosis – It is essential that assessment include demographic data, diagnostic criteria, and personality assessment.
(2) Treatment variables – Individual, group and family counseling and the methods employed, pharmaceutical and nutritional applications, social and vocational skill training, and life changes including health and hobbies.
(3) At home follow-up – This includes substance use, diagnostic criteria re-evaluation, and life changes. Home follow-up also involves verifying what treatment procedures actually took place.

The data from the above three would be used to make improvements to the systems including a better match of subjects and treatments. Indicators, such as relapse rates, would be used to show any improvements over time in the treatment of addiction.

I have recommendations for persons seeking addiction treatment and persons giving treatment. Unlike most books on addiction, I mostly have recommendations for the federal and state governments who are spending millions of dollars on this problem with little concern with results. I emphasize my recommendations for government officials because they can change the current system. I believe it is precisely our medical/psychological approach to addictions that has led to minimal gains over the last 40 years. I believe we need people with Masters of Business degrees (MBA's) to replace physicians and psychologists in charge of government offices on addiction. We also need more statisticians and social scientists (sociologists and anthropologists) working in addictions. Statisticians will only care what works for people who have undergone treatment; not "evidence- based" data from journals or the latest theories on how the brain operates. So far, cultural solutions for addiction have far exceeded what we have achieved through medicine and psychology.

My History

I grew up in Minnesota. Alcoholism is especially high in a state with brutal and depressing winters. My father was a successful professional engineer. In his day he was credited with designing the largest packaging machine. It was for a Canadian lumber company. Unfortunately, he had an alcohol problem for as long as I can remember. He died from alcoholism when I was only 20 years old.

I went on to get a bachelor's degree from the University of Minnesota. The U. of M. was known for dustbowl empiricism. In other words, we care about what works more than fancy theories. My brother is a physicist. Most physicists believe in Dark Matter. Dark Matter explains a lot but has never been measured. That is why I believe, as an empiricist, the concept of Dark Matter is only a holding place and will disappear once someone comes up with something measurable.

Presently, we have good data on how opioids have special receptors in the brain. We know about the brain's pleasure centers and how we use our frontal cortex to make rational decisions and where memories laden with emotion are stored. However, we knew in 1954 that a rat would press a lever that stimulated the nucleus accumbens to the detriment of his wellbeing (Milner & Olds). We were also very familiar with the effects of neurotransmitters such as dopamine and serotonin. This knowledge did not lead to any great accomplishments in treating addictions.

I went on to get my Ph.D. from the University of Texas in psychology. Texas was only second to Harvard in endowment at that time. They had oil money. Consequently, they had the best teachers money can buy. The University of Texas had not one or two but three former American Psychological Association presidents teaching psychology. One of those teachers, Quinn McNemar, I considered as one of my mentors. He not only had his own book in statistics but taught a class on test construction. I learned that psychologists loved tests but rarely did tests help anyone get better.

Right after graduating from the University of Texas I got a job at the psychiatric unit of Brainerd State Hospital. This was a newly created unit at an institution that primarily served the mentally retarded. I had previous worked summers at another state hospital as well a Veterans hospital so I was very familiar with psychiatric patients. The psychiatric unit had a section for the mentally ill and a section for chemical dependency. I was involved with both sections.

Like most hospitals in the 1970's, our program for chemical dependency was based on the 12-step program of Alcoholics Anonymous. Our counselors were all recovering alcoholics. Being fresh out of college I quickly delved into the research literature. Much to my surprise, there was no literature verifying the validity of this approach. My biggest concern was not this lack of validity but why the state of Minnesota would use taxpayers' money to provide a service available for free in the community. Of course, the community provided no inpatient facilities. We were to provide 24 hour per day monitoring and guidance until our clientele were ready to re-enter the community. At that time, they were expected to continue with a local AA group.

It became clear to me and another psychologist at our unit that AA was not sufficient for many of our clients. My colleague decided to work with a small group of some of the more serious cases. We discovered that alcoholics, in general, despise being called mentally ill so we never referred to them with that label even though she ran her group as if they were. Transactional analysis was popular at the time and that became one of her methods.

A few years later, it became clear to me that nearly one-third of our clients were readmissions. It made no sense to me to put them through the 12-step program for a second time. Consequently, I created a program specifically for these people called Time Structuring. This program received an award from The National Institute of

Drug Abuse. I will discuss this program later as we used a method called "exposure and response prevention" that I believe is underused in addiction treatment. Even the 2018 addition from the Harvard Medical School called "Overcoming Addiction" does not mention this therapy.

I also became involved with program evaluation. I wanted to make sure that what we were doing made people better. I discovered that you needed to visit former patients in their homes to get accurate information.

A Few Facts on Opioid Addiction

You all know that opioids have been in the news since the number of deaths have gone up. Between 1999 and 2016, opioid related deaths rose more than four times (*The Week*, March 15, 2019). The United States had about 40,000 opioid related deaths in 2017. New Orleans had 219 accidental drug-related deaths in 2017 (*The Advocate*, April 27, 2018). Drug overdoses for all drugs was over 70,000 in 2017. For the first time in years, the life expectancy for men had gone down.

Today a lot of drug deaths attributed to heroin were actually fentanyl deaths. New Hampshire had 439 drug overdoses in 2015. They believe that up to 70% of these deaths involved fentanyl. In the New Orleans area, it is estimated that about half of opioid deaths involve fentanyl (Newell Normand show, Aug. 20, 2018). The United States had over 28,000 fentanyl related deaths. After two hours on the internet I concluded that roughly 200 milligrams of heroin are fatal, 2 milligrams of fentanyl are fatal, and 20 micrograms of carfentanil are fatal (multiples of 100 at most). Fentanyl has a purpose. It is sometimes used in epidurals for childbirth pain.

The good news is that the number of opioid deaths is likely to diminish for the following reasons:

(1) First responders have naloxone.
(2) Physicians are finally limiting the prescriptions of opioids.
(3) Heroin can be tested for fentanyl with a $2 strip.
(4) It is not a good business practice for dealers to kill their customers.

Physicians are limiting their prescriptions of opioids. As of November 2018, thirty-two states have enacted legislation limiting the number of opioids prescribed to a small number of days, usually seven. The following brand-named medicines are used for pain: Tylenol, Advil, Aleve, Celebrex, Neurontin, Lyrica, Tegretol, Cymbalta, and Pamelor. A study of 240 veterans with back, knee or hip pain did as well on acetaminophen (Tylenol) and ibuprofen (Advil) or Naproxen (Aleve) as on opioids (*JAMA*, Mar. 6, 2018).

One study discovered that 31% of patients between the ages of 16 and 25 were given opioids after their wisdom teeth were pulled. Six percent (6%) went on to abuse opioids. Of those not given opioids, only 0.4% went on to abuse opioids (Erin E. Krebs et al, *JAMA Internal Medicine*, Dec. 2018).

Unfortunately, the states are all going to take credit for the coming reduction in opioid deaths to justify their money. There is a simple test to see if I am right or wrong. If I am correct, the number of opioid related deaths will start dropping in 2019 and will begin to level off at the end of 2020. The states will probably need about a year to put any new plans into effect. Any drop in opioid deaths as the results of these new measures would probably be most prominent beginning in year 2020 and should continue for the next several years. In other words, I predict that the drop in opioid deaths will occur before the states can put their federal money for substance abuse into practice.

I received a response from the Overdose Prevention Coordinator for Florida. Their 27 million dollars "is focused on increasing access to evidence-based prevention, intervention, treatment, and recovery support services for individuals with opioid use disorders who are uninsured, underinsured, or indigent. The majority of the funding is being spent to expand access to medication-assisted treatment (MAT) services for individuals with opioid use disorder." I do not doubt that people will be helped with this money. However, when the money runs out, they are back to square one. Using the money to put a system in place, such as the one I recommend, would continue to produce gains.

According to the Associated Press, March 2018, the United States Government is spending 4.6 billion dollars in 2018 on the opioid crisis. Louisiana was given 24 million dollars. Florida, home of old people and pain clinics, was once the opioid capital of the United States. Many of the pain clinics have been shut down and a pharmaceutical company was taken to court. Florida is not the only one responsible for **not creating a system** to improve the treatment of addiction. The federal government makes no stipulations requiring that states receiving money to fight the opioid epidemic do any treatment follow-up studies assessing relapse rates.

The National Council on Alcoholism and Drug Dependency estimates that over 23 million Americans are addicted to alcohol and other drugs. Two-thirds of persons in our prisons have substance abuse problems. The Substance Abuse and Mental Health Services Administration (SAMHSA) estimates that addiction treatment is a $35 billion per year business.

The National Institute on Drug Abuse (NIDA) states the relapse rate for addiction is between 40% to 60%. They say this is because drug addiction is a chronic illness like diabetes, hypertension, and asthma. In the article that compares drug abuse to diabetes, hypertension and asthma, it says "studies indicate that less than 30% of patients with adult-onset asthma, hypertension, or diabetes adhere to prescribed diet and/or behavioral changes that are designed to increase functional status and reduce risk factors for recurrence of the disorders." (McLellan et al, *JAMA*, 2000, 284(13)). Perhaps these three illnesses are not chronic at all. They only appear to be chronic illnesses because patients will not adhere to treatment.

Given that people with hypertension do not seek out stressful situations and asthmatics do not seek out smoke filled rooms, diabetes 2 is the only comparable chronic illness to addiction. Some people with type 2 diabetes do go into remission with weight loss, proper diet, exercise and sleep. However, every addict has the possibility of remission. Furthermore, "To diagnose type 2 diabetes, you'll be given a: Glycated hemoglobin (A1C) test. This blood test indicates your average blood sugar level for the past two to three months. ... An A1C level of 6.5 percent or higher on two separate tests indicates you have diabetes" (Mayo Clinic Sep. 2018). There currently is no medical test for drug abuse. Can you imagine the difficulty of diagnosing type 2 diabetes with a questionnaire?

According to William R. Miller and Kathleen M. Carroll, "Most people who recover from drug problems do so on their own, without formal treatment" (*Rethinking Substance Abuse*, p. 295). How many other chronic illnesses can you say this about?

More important than what NIDA says about addiction is what they do not say. If drug abuse was going down over the years or if the treatment of drug abuse was becoming more and more successful, do you think the NIDA would be showing charts of various chronic illnesses? I cannot find any charts of addiction relapse rates over the years. To the best of my knowledge it remains between 50% and 60%. Lower percentages are possible, especially if the addict's job is on the line.

Lloyd Sederer, M.D. wrote "The Addiction Solution" (Scribner, 2018). This man was once the chief medical officer for the New York State Office of Mental Health. He has written several books and hundreds of articles. As I see it, you can only claim an addiction solution by presenting a treatment program that consistently beats a relapse rate of 50%. (Note: The publisher might have chosen the title.) He presents a single study on relapse rates. A three-and-a-half-year follow-up on opioid dependent people who were given an opioid replacement showed 50% of them to be clean at 18 months and 60% at the end of the study. Clearly this is a promising study but hardly justifies a whole book.

Adam Bisaga, M.D. wrote "Overcoming Opioid Addiction" (The Experiment, 2018) In his book he refers to "many studies" showing the superiority of the Medically Assisted Therapy (MAT) for the addictions. Unfortunately, he does not list any relapse rates for this method. Of course, the term "medically assisted" implies other unmentioned therapies were employed. To say that using multiple means to cure addiction is the best approach tells nothing.

Let me add that I am actually a believer in giving addicts buprenorphine or some other opioid agonist or antagonist. How long any specific person should take these drugs, however, is unknown. I also supported Antabuse for alcoholics in the 1970's when few people did. However, I would not be writing this book if I thought we were even close to the successful treatment of addiction.

With a myriad of books by professionals and former addicts on addiction as well as thousands of studies on addiction in over 20 journals, why is there no definitive evidence as to whether we are getting better at treating addiction? With most schools running drug prevention programs, why is there no evidence of drug use steadily diminishing? In fact, the use of opioids and other drugs has increased from 2002 through 2017. Smoking has gone down but about 37% of 12th graders reported vaping in 2018, compared with 28% percent in 2017 (newsinhealth.nih.gov/2019/02/vaping). Note: smoking is the exception which I will discuss later under "Cultural Considerations".

My answer as to why we do not know if treatment for addiction is improving is because we do not have a system in place to continually monitor, modify and assess addiction treatment programs. These systems can only be put in place by government. The federal government has allocated about one-half a billion dollars to the opioid crisis. Unfortunately, to my knowledge, none of this money has been earmarked for the states to create such a system.

Brief History of Opioids

Nearly every book on addiction gives something on history so I will be brief. During the Civil War the Union dispensed about 10 million opium pills to soldiers. In the late nineteenth century, doctors prescribed opium for menstrual cramps. "Before 1900, the typical opiate addict in America was an upper-class or middle-class white woman" (Smithsonian.com, Jan. 4, 2018).

Prohibition encouraged women to drink as drinking was no longer primarily in saloons. Prohibition also increased the use of heroin. Coke Cola had cocaine. Sigmund Freud was addicted to it. Crack cocaine became popular in the 1980's.

It has been said that Nixon started the war on drugs to take people's minds off of the Viet Nam war. His primary concern was the use of heroin. The biggest pocket of heroin users were poor black people in New York City. Allegedly, Nixon was not worried about people who were dying of heroin. He was concerned with them robbing people to support their habit. Evidently, Nixon did not like hippies so he added marijuana to the war on drugs (*Smoke and Mirrors* by Dan Baum, 1996).

In the 1990's pain became the fifth vital sign. This led to more physicians prescribing pain medicine including opioids. This concept was dropped in 2016 as opioid use flourished. According to a 2012 National Health Interview Survey, 11.2% of adults are in chronic pain and 17.6 percent have experienced severe pain. Scientists are working to find an objective measure of pain using brain scans and pupillary responses.

More recently, we determined that there are opioid receptors in the brain and that there are people prone to addiction. However, many teenagers seem to be addicted to their electronic devises. No doubt cell phone addiction is rising. Four large studies show that twice as many heavy users of electronic devices (over two hours per day) are depressed or distressed compared with light users (*Time*, April, 2019). At this time, gambling is the only official (DSM-5) behavioral addiction. I expect computer gaming to be next.

The definition of maturity is the ability to forego immediate pleasures for long-term satisfaction (i.e. go to school, get a job, work hard). These traits are strongly related to social class and the expectations of the child and parents. With more people addicted to their cell phones and social media, can we expect more people to choose the instant gratification that is available in drugs?

Diagnosis and Referral

Most books on addiction go out of their way to emphasize that addiction is a disease/illness. One definition of a disease is a disorder of structure or function in a person that produces specific signs or symptoms or that affects a specific location and is not simply a direct result of physical injury.

Is obesity a disease/illness? Obesity is certainly a factor in diabetes and heart disease. Some people think that eating something sweet only makes you want more. Obese people even have brains different from normal people. "Compared to healthy weight individuals, the obese adults had reduced gray matter volume in several brain regions, including the hippocampus, prefrontal cortex, and other subcortical regions. ... These findings add to a growing body of literature demonstrating that obesity is associated with decreases in brain and cognitive health, which can be linked to mechanisms involving peripheral and central metabolic dysfunction ... While somewhat variable across studies, diet-induced weight loss improved attention and executive control" (Stillman et al, *Aging Neuroscience*, 2017, 9 (115)). Similar to drug addiction, some treatments for obesity are medical (e.g. prescription medicines and surgery) while others are not (e.g., diet, exercise and environmental changes).

Many of the recent books on drug addiction say that if only people realized that it is an illness, addicts would be treated better. Several authors make a heartfelt plea to look at drug abuse as if it were a disease like cancer. Before they put too much effort into this endeavor, they should consider the following facts:

1) People have been saying this about mental illness for over 50 years.
2) We are one of the few countries in the world that has never had a woman leader.
3) Minorities believe that white males are favored for the top positions.
4) More than 70% of the LGBT community believe churches are unfriendly (2013 survey).
5) Children are being bullied; some have even committed suicide.
6) Many of the disabled believe they are treated as if they were invisible.
7) We have a maximum-security prison where people are held in solitary confinement for 23 hours per day and the Supreme Court does not consider this to be "cruel and unusual" punishment.

8) We have something called "Not guilty by reason of insanity". Evidently mass murderers are sane. If you consider insanity as not being able to distinguish right from wrong, then all terrorists who kill infidels would fall under this definition. Only about .0025 of all homicides get this verdict.
9) One out of three people are obese. Look at people on television and people elected to office. Are one out of three of these people obese?
10) Ugly women cannot get a job on Fox News or anywhere else. A study was done in Italy were 10,000 identical resumes were sent out with different pictures of the applicant attached. The callback rate was 54% for attractive women whereas the callback rate was 7% for the unattractive women (*Business Insider*, 2013, Sept. 13).

My point is that there is a long line of people who get no respect.

I remember when we wanted to call drunks "alcoholics" (an illness) to remove the stigma so people would get help. Today, hardly anyone talks about drunks. Unfortunately, the word alcoholic has become increasingly pejorative. Furthermore, by claiming alcoholism was a disease, we just made Alcoholics Anonymous appear to be a sham. By insisting that drug addiction is an illness because its ingestion affects the brain, how is that going to affect the thousands of people who will soon be addicted to computer games, their cell phones and the internet? There is no question that drugs like heroin affect the brain in ways that lead to addiction. However, that is only half of the story. I have yet to see a study as to how the brains of people who use heroin on a regular basis without getting into trouble differ from those who do.

As previously mentioned, many people point out that mental illness is a legitimate disease. The official list of mental illnesses is in a manual called the Diagnostic and Statistical Manual (DSM). We are presently on number 5. The first edition came out in 1952. It had 106 categories. By 1994 (DSM-4) the categories shot up to 297. Do we have over twice as many people with mental illness today than in the 1950's?

Sadly, the DSM has the word "statistical" in it. Find me a Ph.D. statistician who doesn't think the DSM is a joke? Find me a study that shows that clinicians reliably agree on a person's diagnosis. Based on the DSM there are 256 different ways to have Borderline Personality Disorder (Abion et al, *Comprehensive Psychiatry*, 2012, 54). There are 636,120 different ways to have Post Traumatic Stress Syndrome (Galatzer-Levy et al, *Personal Psychological Science Journal*, 2013, 8). In 1952, we had 21 personality disorders. By the year 2000, only 3 or the 21 remained unchanged -paranoid, schizoid, and antisocial (*The Harvard Mental Health Letter*, 2000, Mar.). Another study of 936 hospitalized patients followed for seven years found that only half of those eventually diagnosed with schizophrenia began with that diagnosis (*The Harvard Mental Health Letter*, 1998, July).

As a statistician and behaviorist, I suggest we throw out the DSM and instead create a manual with a list of behaviors such as loss of appetite, believing your mind is being controlled, difficulty getting to sleep, feeling unloved, craving attention, etc. Then we have to determine whether clinicians can reliably agree that a person demonstrates the behavior(s) in question. By repeated measurements over time, statisticians will be able to determine which behaviors cluster together, which behaviors are likely to change over time, and which behaviors are most likely to change given some intervention such as counseling or medications.

In actual fact, DSM diagnoses are already made up of a list of behaviors. The problem is that the behaviors are grouped before a statistical analysis says they belong together. Statisticians use a statistical method called factor analysis to determine actual groupings.

We need to convince insurance companies to allow everyone so many hours of clinical assistance such as counseling without needing an official diagnosis. As I see it, insurance companies are one of the primary reasons we have diagnoses. I see a future where everyone is seen as unique and we begin to veer away from assuming a general diagnosis calls for a general treatment.

I realize that many people are trying hard to remove the stigma of addiction by saying it is a disease. Some people believe that Hitler was a paranoid schizophrenic. If I could convince you of this, would you feel sorry for him?

If we should be sympathetic to someone with a disease, then it is acceptable to despise and punish people who simply made bad choices? Furthermore, children who grew up in orphanages, children of alcoholics and children who were regularly beaten do not have a disease. Should we treat them with less sympathy than someone with cancer? Ugly people who are perfectly healthy with good skills and personality are discriminated against every day.

Philosophers have debated for years whether we have free will or whether we are simply victims of genetics and environment. The simple solution to this conundrum is to **treat everyone with respect and dignity**. Thinking you need a diagnosis to be treated with respect is stupid! If two people agree that it would be best if one of them no longer relied on a certain substance, we only need to know what methods work best to achieve this goal. When someone else's behavior negatively affects you, you have to decide how to minimize their effect on you. If a person you know wants to engage in self-destructive behavior, you have the option of avoiding them, trying to dissuade the person, or seeking professional help to intervene.

The National Institute on Drug Abuse states "Addiction is defined as a chronic, relapsing disorder characterized by compulsive drug seeking, continued use despite harmful consequences, and long-lasting changes in the brain. It is considered both a complex brain disorder and a mental illness. Addiction is the most severe form of a full spectrum of substance use disorders, and is a **medical illness** caused by repeated misuse of a substance or substances."

Remember Bernie Madoff? He appeared to be addicted to money. He never had enough. Bernie Madoff might someday write a book about stealing. However, for every rich man addicted to money, there are thirty men who steal because they are poor. Perhaps for everyone addicted (via genetics) to drugs, there are thirty people who take drugs simply because they are miserable.

Various authors often make it clear that their intent is to alleviate guilt by inferring that addicts are not weak people with no will power. Do these same people disparage Narcotics Anonymous (NA)? The first step of NA is admitting you are powerless over your addiction. Isn't "powerless" the same as "weak"? Of course, the other side of the coin is that people can claim they are helpless because they have an illness (addiction).

Let's first deal with the word "chronic". I was taught that an alcoholic is never cured but an alcoholic can be a recovering alcoholic. According to one dictionary, a chronic illness is "having an illness persisting for a long time or constantly recurring". Is the common cold a chronic illness? Is the flu a chronic illness? Is cancer a chronic illness? If I often tell a lie, am I a chronic liar?

Clearly the word "chronic" is too vague to be very useful. I prefer the word "predisposed". Predisposed is defined as to "make someone liable or inclined to a specified attitude, action, or condition." I believe that some people are predisposed to gain weight, have heart trouble or become addicted. (Hopefully, no one is predisposed to become a liar.) It is my guess that when we have a better handle on genetics and upbringing, we will know which people are indeed predisposed to become addicted. Clearly, people who do not respond well to alcohol, as is true of some Asians, are not predisposed to become alcoholics.

People like to refer to themselves as "recovering" addicts or alcoholics. If I periodically get colds, does that make me a "recovering" person between bouts? There is a problem with saying a drug addict or an alcoholic is one for life. If someone treated for alcoholism goes back to moderate drinking, you are forced to say that either the person was not a "true" alcoholic or that his drinking will eventually create a problem. I was always weary of labeling someone under the age of thirty as an alcoholic. Many a college binge drinker changes after college, marriage and employment. This does not mean the person did not have a drinking problem while in college. It only means he is not destined to be a lifelong alcoholic. On the other hand, I have no problem with calling a man over forty with a long history of alcohol abuse an alcoholic. One author of a book I read does not like the term "addict". He prefers to be a person with "substance use disorder". I do not see this phrase as ever becoming popular. Furthermore, would you know what I was talking about if I said I know a teenager with "Internet use disorder"?

I also believe that it is possible that some time in the future we might be better able to diagnose addiction by neurological testing or measuring brain function. However, without one's genome and personal history, we may never be able to say with any degree of certainty that an individual will always be predisposed to addiction. We presently know that poverty, stress and early trauma predisposed a person to addiction but we cannot say that this person will always be that way.

It is said that when sick people see a physician and are given a medical label of an illness, they feel better. Let's suppose you came to me for psychotherapy. In order for your insurance to pay for this, I need to give you an official diagnosis. So, I put down "Borderline Personality Disorder". Everything is going smoothly with our sessions until one day, out of curiosity, you want to know your diagnosis. You go home and look it up on the internet and this is what you see as the symptoms of this diagnosis on a National Institute of Mental Health website:

- Efforts to avoid real or imagined abandonment, such as rapidly initiating intimate (physical or emotional) relationships or cutting off communication with someone in anticipation of being abandoned
- A pattern of intense and unstable relationships with family, friends, and loved ones, often swinging from extreme closeness and love (idealization) to extreme dislike or anger (devaluation)
- Distorted and unstable self-image or sense of self
- Impulsive and often dangerous behaviors, such as spending sprees, unsafe sex, substance abuse, reckless driving, and binge eating. **Please note:** If these behaviors occur primarily during a period of elevated mood or energy, they may be signs of a mood disorder—not borderline personality disorder
- Self-harming behavior, such as cutting
- Recurring thoughts of suicidal behaviors or threats

- Intense and highly changeable moods, with each episode lasting from a few hours to a few days
- Chronic feelings of emptiness
- Inappropriate, intense anger or problems controlling anger
- Difficulty trusting, which is sometimes accompanied by irrational fear of other people's intentions
- Feelings of dissociation, such as feeling cut off from oneself, seeing oneself from outside one's body, or feelings of unreality

Do you think that by knowing you have this official diagnosis you are going to feel better?

The internet is kind when it comes to the definition of addiction. The *International Journal of Environmental Research and Public Health* (Oct. 2011) says "The definition of addiction is explored. Elements of addiction derived from a literature search that uncovered 52 studies include: (a) engagement in the behavior to achieve appetitive effects, (b) preoccupation with the behavior, (c) temporary satiation, (d) loss of control, and (e) suffering negative consequences."

All definitions of addiction mention negative or harmful consequences. Perhaps people would not be so endeared with this diagnosis if they mentioned that some of the negative consequences included:

(1) Dying from an overdose
(2) Becoming a dealer and getting shot or going to prison
(3) Becoming a prostitute
(4) Being physically or sexually abused
(5) Stealing from friends and relatives

(6) Lying about your activities
(7) Losing your job
(8) Losing your spouse and children
(9) Medical problems such as HIV or hepatitis
(10) Other problems from a living style of poor nutrition and lack of exercise

How do I feel about diagnosis? I am a behaviorist. I don't need a general label. I need to know what specific behaviors need to be changed. Labels are generalizations. Some are clearly better (i.e., more predictive) than others. If you tell me you are a conservative, can I assume you probably drive a hybrid to conserve our natural resources? Given our 22 trillion-dollar debt, fiscal conservatives must be a rarity in the United States. If I were to create a measure of how liberal or conservative people are, would my graph of these measurements be bimodal (two peaks)? My point is that I don't know what liberal or conservative means, but I can measure how much different people give to charity in absolute dollars and percent of income. I can measure which government programs a person would like to support.

Some labels might be too inclusive. Can you say you believe in states rights and still support a federal law against gay marriage? Can you say a woman is in charge of her own body but be against prostitution?

The fact that schizophrenia is a brain disease determined primarily by genetics does not alter my interest in behavior. I have no problem with using chemistry (psychotropics, tranquilizers, opioid agonists, etc.) to alter behavior. Consider the following examples:

(1) Alex has been a professional musician for many years. Most of this time he has used drugs including heroin. Alex is concerned that his drug use is getting in the way of performing.
(2) Cindy is a seventeen-year-old who is on heroin. She dropped out of school and is living with an older couple who are also users. Cindy brings in money as a prostitute. Her parents have begged her to come to me for help which she has reluctantly agreed to.
(3) Robert was sent to me by a drug court because he is a first-time offender. He is in his late twenties and is a small-time dealer as well as a user.

Do I treat these people alike because they are all opioid drug addicts? Certainly not. Alex needs harm reduction. Although we can talk about abstinence, it is unlikely he would follow it. Alex needs to develop a plan of limited/controlled drug use that he can actually maintain. Should he fail at this, we could discuss more serious measures.

Cindy needs family counseling as well as one-to-one counseling. The family and Cindy need to find agreement on acceptable behaviors and consequences. I need to deal with Cindy on life style changes as well as dealing with her thoughts and emotions (i.e., cognitive therapy).

For Robert, I need to go back to the court and tell them that he needs to be in a standard addiction treatment program with people who know a lot more about his situation than I do and can deal with his objections.

Although it is a cliché to "deal with the whole person", it is difficult to separate the influence of heredity, personality and environment for most problems including addictions. Here is another example.

Many scientists, including myself, believe the issue of how much of any behavior is genetics and how much is the environment is often misconstrued. Let me take the analogy of a prize-winning cake. Is it the ingredients or the process that make a cake a winner? Suppose we discover that baking the cake a few minutes too short or too long takes it out of contention. Does that prove that the process is critical? What if just a little too much butter ruins the cake? Does that show how important the ingredients are? If most of a cake is flour and water but a touch of cinnamon separates the first prize from the second prize, which ingredient is more important? It is perfectly reasonable to study genetics, environment, and their interaction. However, the best answer as to what makes a prize-winning cake is "everything" – *including the judges who ate it.*

How do you choose between inpatient and outpatient? Usually the treatment center makes this decision. Do you trust them when inpatient treatment costs several times more than outpatient? Likewise, group therapy at $50 per person makes the center $500 with ten people in the group and one therapist. Individual therapy makes the center $150 with one therapist. Some addicts/alcoholics recover on their own (school of hard knocks plus friends and relatives, clergy, etc.). That is why I believe <u>no one should do both diagnosis and treatment</u>.

Unfortunately, Mental Health Centers do this all the time. I would guess that very few people who show up at a Mental Health Center are told that they do not need any counseling.

The state needs to set up diagnostic centers for mental health and addiction that operate independently from treatment. Independent means that these diagnostic centers cannot be a part of, or even near a state-run treatment center. The state should provide this service from federal and state monies. By not being in the treatment business, these recommendations would be unbiased. These same diagnostic centers would include all psychiatric illnesses.

In the best of all worlds, I believe that the states should be getting out of the treatment business as they expand diagnosis and follow-up. The poor will always need to be subsidized for serious problems. The state does not need treatment centers for addiction anymore than they need state hospitals for cancer patients.

It is common for addicts to have co-occurring diagnoses. Approximately 53 percent of all drug addicts and 37 percent of alcoholics also have a mental health disorder (National Alliance on Mental Illness, May, 2016). Some of the more popular co-occurring diagnoses include ADHD (20%), Anti-social personality disorder (18%), and borderline personality (16%). Several experts question whether most addiction treatment centers can adequately handle co-occurring psychiatric disorders. Nearly all of the experts agree that co-occurring psychiatric disorders need to be treated concurrently with addiction.

Drug addicts and alcoholics might also have related illnesses. Drug addicts who use needles are also more likely to have hepatitis C (65%) and 8% of persons with HIV are drug users (NIDA, May, 2015). Alcoholics are more likely to have cirrhosis of the liver, cardiomyopathy, pancreatitis, and even dementia. Addicts, in general, might have physical problems related to poor nutrition, lack of exercise, and poor sleep. According to the Harvard Medical School, "The relationship between poor quality sleep and worsening pain has important implications for individuals experiencing both acute and chronic pain. More or better sleep may lessen the pain that they are experiencing" (Posted February 18, 2019).

The Diagnostic and Statistical Manual (DSM-5) consists of 23 questions in 13 diagnostic categories. If a person scores high on a diagnostic category such as depression, he or she is asked additional questions such as weight gain or loss, feelings of fatigue, and difficulty concentrating. The category of substance abuse has 11 additional questions.

The DSM-5 asks the following questions to determine substance abuse:

Criteria for Substance Use Disorders

1. Taking the substance in larger amounts or for longer than you're meant to.
2. Wanting to cut down or stop using the substance but not managing to.
3. Spending a lot of time getting, using, or recovering from use of the substance.

4. Cravings and urges to use the substance.
5. Not managing to do what you should at work, home, or school because of substance use.
6. Continuing to use, even when it causes problems in relationships.
7. Giving up important social, occupational, or recreational activities because of substance use.
8. Using substances again and again, even when it puts you in danger.
9. Continuing to use, even when you know you have a physical or psychological problem that could have been caused or made worse by the substance.
10. Needing more of the substance to get the effect you want (tolerance).
11. Development of withdrawal symptoms, which can be relieved by taking more of the substance.

Two or three symptoms indicate a mild substance use disorder; four or five symptoms indicate a moderate substance use disorder, and six or more symptoms indicate a severe substance use disorder.

As I see it, these are only guidelines. If someone only met criteria "1" because the person had to be taken to the emergency room to be resuscitated, would he or she be sent home for not meeting the official criteria of addiction?

One of the reasons I like behavioral checklists is that <u>this same checklist can be used on follow-up by someone who does not know what the original assessment was.</u>

The Addiction Severity Index (ASI)can be used for an in-depth evaluation. According to a National Institute of Health government website, "The ASI is a semi-structured interview designed to address seven potential problem areas in substance-abusing patients: medical status, employment and support, drug use, alcohol use, legal status, family/social status, and psychiatric status. In 1 hour, a skilled interviewer can gather information on recent (past 30 days) and lifetime problems in all of the problem areas. The ASI provides an overview of problems related to substance abuse, rather than focusing on any single area."

At the other extreme is the "30 Day" measure of addiction. This works for any addiction whether substance abuse, cell phone addiction, or watching sports. The subject is told that if he or she can go 30 days without the thing they crave, they are not addicted. The good news is that is test does not take 30 days; it only takes one minute. Why? Because an addicted person will refuse to give the 30 days a try.

Of course, referral centers would normally collect a standard set of demographic data including sex, age, socioeconomic level (i.e., income and educational level), family/marital status, occupation, and interests and hobbies. Furthermore, the assessment should include one's medical history and any previous diagnoses and traumas.

I believe it is helpful to have a significant other with the person during the initial interview. This significant other can be a spouse, relative, neighbor, or friend. Sometimes it takes another party to clarify exactly the behaviors that need to be changed. Even with drug abuse, everyone will need to make more behavioral changes beyond no drug use or reduced/safer use. Not all of these target behaviors are going to focus on the negative. Many will be positive lifestyle changes to both replace drug use and to provide long term health and personal growth and satisfaction.

A psychological/personality assessment is necessary to determine if substance abuse clients can be matched to treatment programs best suited for them. I would personally recommend the Minnesota Multiphasic Personality Inventory (MMPI) as well as the Big Five Personality Test.

The MMPI is based on whether you answer the questions similar to those in the following diagnostic categories (https://psychcentral.com):

1. **Hypochondriasis** (Hs) – The Hypochondriasis scale tapes a wide variety of vague and nonspecific complaints about bodily functioning. These complaints tend to focus on the abdomen and back, and they persist in the face of negative medical tests. There are two primary factors that this subscale measures — poor physical health and gastrointestinal difficulties. The scale contains 32 items.
2. **Depression** (D) – The Depression scale measures clinical depression, which is characterized by poor morale, lack of hope in the future, and a general dissatisfaction with one's life. The scale contains 57 items.
3. **Hysteria** (Hy) – The Hysteria scale primarily measures five components — poor physical health, shyness, cynicism, headaches and neuroticism. The subscale contains 60 items.

4. **Psychopathic Deviate** (Pd) – The Psychopathic Deviate scale measures general social maladjustment and the absence of strongly pleasant experiences. The items on this scale tap into complaints about family and authority figures in general, self-alienation, social alienation and boredom. The scale contains 50 items.
5. **Masculinity/Femininity** (Mf) – The Masculinity/Femininity scale measures interests in vocations and hobbies, aesthetic preferences, activity-passivity and personal sensitivity. It measures in a general sense how rigidly a person conforms to very stereotypical masculine or feminine roles. The scale contains 56 items.
6. **Paranoia** (Pa) – The Paranoia scale primarily measures interpersonal sensitivity, moral self-righteousness and suspiciousness. Some of the items used to score this scale are clearly psychotic in that they acknowledge the existence of paranoid and delusional thoughts. This scale has 40 items.
7. **Psychasthenia** (Pt) -The Psychasthenia scale is intended to measure a person's inability to resist specific actions or thoughts, regardless of their maladaptive nature. "Psychasthenia" is an old term used to describe what we now call obsessive-compulsive disorder (OCD), or having obsessive-compulsive thoughts and behaviors. This scale also taps into abnormal fears, self-criticisms, difficulties in concentration and guilt feelings. This scale contains 48 items.
8. **Schizophrenia** (Sc) – The Schizophrenia scale measures bizarre thoughts, peculiar perceptions, social alienation, poor familial relationships, difficulties in concentration and impulse control, lack of deep interests, disturbing question of self-worth and self-identity, and sexual difficulties. This scale has 78 items, more than any other scale on the test.

9. **Hypomania** (Ma) – The Hypomania scale is intended to measure milder degrees of excitement, characterized by an elated but unstable mood, psychomotor excitement (e.g., shaky hands) and flight of ideas (e.g., an unstoppable string of ideas). The scale taps into overactivity — both behaviorally and cognitively — grandiosity, irritability and egocentricity. This scale contains 46 items.
10. **Social Introversion** (Si) – The Social Introversion scale measures the social introversion and extroversion of a person. A person who is a social introvert is uncomfortable in social interactions and typically withdraws from such interactions whenever possible. They may have limited social skills, or simply prefer to be alone or with a small group of friends. This scale has 69 items.

The MMPI is not a valid measure of a person's psychopathology or behavior if the person taking the test does so in a way that is not honest or frank. A person may decide, for whatever reasons, to overreport (exaggerate) or underreport (deny) the behavior being assessed by the test. Consequently, the MMPI contains four validity scales designed to measure a person's test-taking attitude and approach to the test.

There exists a wealth of data on how MMPI profiles relate to personality and behavioral tendencies.

The Big Five measures (www.123test.com):

- **Openness**
- **Conscientiousness**

- **Extraversion**
- **Agreeableness**
- **Neuroticism**

- Openness - People who like to learn new things and enjoy new experiences usually score high in openness. Openness includes traits like being insightful and imaginative and having a wide variety of interests.
- Conscientiousness - People that have a high degree of conscientiousness are reliable and prompt. Traits include being organized, methodic, and thorough.
- Extraversion - Extraverts get their energy from interacting with others, while introverts get their energy from within themselves. Extraversion includes the traits of energetic, talkative, and assertive.
- Agreeableness - These individuals are friendly, cooperative, and compassionate. People with low agreeableness may be more distant. Traits include being kind, affectionate, and sympathetic.
- Neuroticism - Neuroticism is also sometimes called Emotional Stability. This dimension relates to one's emotional stability and degree of negative emotions.

People that score high on neuroticism often experience emotional instability and negative emotions. Traits include being moody and tense.

Diagnosis will help individualize a person's treatment. For example, if the person is highly stressed, they might recommend a treatment center with meditation and yoga, or even one with a religious orientation.

Several studies indicate the effects on long-term drug use on the brain. Consequently, when dealing with drug addiction, a test of neurological/cognitive functioning would be desirable. These tests measure things like:

(1) Memory – including recognition, working memory, short-term memory, and non-verbal memory
(2) Attention and concentration
(3) Reaction time
(4) Planning and executive function
(5) Hand-eye coordination

Unfortunately, a typical neuropsychological evaluation takes approximately six hours. Unlike personality tests, a short test of cognitive functioning would be ideal for a pre-treatment and post-treatment evaluation. Some cognitive functioning tests are available over the Internet. Perhaps some time in the future, we will be able to do a quick and inexpensive assessment of neurotransmitters such as dopamine and serotonin.

In the future I expect referral counselors will enter information about the potential client into a computer.

This will include demographic data, history, personality and neurological testing. The computer will then show this person's chances of being sober/clean in one year. For example, it might indicate those chances are between 32% and 45% (a 90% confidence interval meaning that 9 out of 10 times the person will fall in this range). The referral counselor will then do "what if" scenarios. In other words, what are the client's chances of being drug free given Narcotics Anonymous attendance, Medication-Assisted Treatment, outpatient counseling, starting a new hobby, etc. It may be that finding a job does the most to improve his chances for sobriety. Expect diminishing returns. Adding a fourth treatment/behavior to the list might do very little to lessen his chances of a relapse. As more client follow-up data is entered into the computer, the better these predictions will become.

Why should the states be the primary source for referrals to addiction treatment centers? Presently, most people go to Google. Unfortunately, addiction treatment centers all sound the same. "They promise comparable recovery rates, therapy modules, and creature comforts" (Ryan Hampton, *American Fix*, 2018). Only recently, in 2017, did Google stop the practice of allowing addiction treatment centers to pay for a favorable placement (ibid). People, such as those on television ads, are handsomely paid for referrals. Who else but the state has the resources to insure minimum competency? Who else can investigate possible fraud? With the states doing treatment follow-up, they will only get better over time at providing referrals.

Measuring Progress

I have worked with the mentally ill and the addicted. It is difficult to assess the severity of many mental illnesses such as schizophrenia. Schizophrenia has many symptoms such as hallucinations, paranoid thinking, inappropriate social behavior, unusual thought patterns, catatonia and lack of affect. Is the lack of emotion more or less serious than an inappropriate emotional response? Is a person who avoids social interaction more or less schizophrenic than a person who hears imaginary voices?

In 2016 the Surgeon General created a seven-chapter book on *Facing Addiction in America*. Chapter 4 dealt with principles of effective treatment, evidence-based treatment, and emerging treatment technologies. They refer to recovery <u>rate</u> as "the proportion of patients who have graduated and remained abstinent." However, recovery itself refers to much more than that. The Substance Abuse and Mental Health Services Administration (SAMHSA) defines recovery as a process of change through which individuals improve their health and wellness, live a self-directed life, and strive to reach their full potential."

Obviously, recovery is difficult to measure. The good news is that it is easy to measure recovery rate in overcoming one's addictions. Abstinence is the standard for the addictions. Certainly, there are other signs of progress such as using less or no longer driving a vehicle when under the influence. Furthermore, a person might have had a single slip and then continue to be sober. Chances are, that if a treatment center has a lot of clients that stayed sober/clean for a year, they probably also had several other clients who made some other sort of progress.

The gold standard for the treatment of addictions is the percent of clients who go one year sober/clean.

Therefore assessing the progress we have made with treating addictions over the years should be easy. We simply plot the percentages of persons leaving treatment remaining sober/clean for each year in the last 50 years.

Would you like to see the results? So would I. I have been contacting treatment centers off and on over many years. The data does not exist. The American Society of Addictive Medicine says the relapse rate for drug addiction is 40% to 60%. They do not say how long this has been true.

A key finding of a report from the National Institute of Drug Abuse (NIDA), July 2014 is: "Well-supported scientific evidence shows that substance use disorders can be effectively treated, with recurrence rates no higher than those for other chronic illnesses." Evidently, they believe a relapse rate of 50% indicates "effective" treatment.

Very few studies give the relapse rate for opioid addiction. A 2002 study followed 242 persons for 12 months following opioid treatment. They found a relapse rate of 60%. (Society for the Study of Addiction).

Another study done in 2010 had a relapse rate of 91% (99 out of 109 patients) for a six-week inpatient program for opioid addiction. Over half of these (59%) relapsed in the first month. (*Irish Med J.* 2010, 103(6)).

Surprisingly, a study in India based on 466 subjects had only a 32% rate of relapse for users of heroin over a year. (*J Addict* 2016, Sept. 18).

There are even fewer studies on adolescent substance abuse. One review said the "Average rate of sustained abstinence after treatment is 38% (range 30-55) at 6 months and 32% at 12 months (range 14-47)" (*Clinical Psychology: Science and Practice,* June 2000).

If the standard for addiction success is being "clean" for a year, it is easy to become discouraged over the low success rate for an addiction. However, a relapse does not imply that no gains were made in treatment but does reset the clock. The relapse rate for smokers is about 88 percent. Still, many a smoker has eventually quit after several tries. There exists some evidence that opioid users who persist for several years have a reasonable chance of remission. The secret to success is perseverance.

One issue unique to drug addiction is that many addicts use more than one drug. Suppose a heroin user takes methadone and no longer uses heroin. If the person still uses cocaine is that person a failure? What if he smokes marijuana, is he a partial failure? In the best of all worlds, follow-up would test for a variety of drugs.

Relapse rates cannot be just for those that finish the program. Unless a person is in treatment under a court order, the job of every counselor or program includes motivating people to stick with the program. Based on 34 studies (2,340 patients) of psychosocial interventions for substance use disorders, one-third of the patients dropped out before treatment completion (*American J. of Psychiatry* 2008 Feb; 165(2)). The percent of clients who make it through a whole program is an important statistic but does not change the gold standard. The practice of Motivational Interviewing is intended to encourage addicts to continue to seek sobriety.

The bottom line is that we do not know if we have been making progress in treating addiction over the last 40 years. We are not even sure what the expected success rates are for the present treatment of opioid abuse.

Types of Treatment

The various treatments for persons with addiction include several standard therapies:

1. Cognitive therapy focuses on how one's beliefs and use of words color one's perceptions. Clients learn to challenge and reframe their beliefs to increase their power over addiction.
2. Contingency Management primarily uses rewards to increase the frequency of behaviors that reduce or are incompatible with addiction behaviors. A subset of Contingency Management uses vouchers

that can be turned in for various rewards such as food or movies when clients do things such as attend meetings and produce drug free urine tests.

3. The Twelve Step Program is based on admitting you are powerless to overcome your addiction alone but by surrendering to a higher power and relying on group support as well as a sponsor, you can be a recovering addict/alcoholic. Twelve Step Facilitation prepares a person for the Twelve Step Program.
4. Motivation Interviewing/Enhancement Therapy helps clients create healthy goals and activities when they are ready that will allow them to be self-sufficient without relying on drugs.
5. Family and group therapy use peer pressure to change a client's behavior. Family therapy might also involve altering the family dynamics if the behaviors of family members are detrimental to the client.

In addition to the above therapeutic methods, there are support services such as helping a person find employment, a place to live or medical/dental aid. Furthermore, there are supplemental therapies such as religion, yoga, music, art and exercise.

In the 1970's I created the following list of treatment programs for alcoholism:

(1) Alcoholics Anonymous – 12 step work, peer pressure, modeling

(2) Psychotherapy/Counseling

(A) Analytic-Intensive (B) Nondirective-Supportive

(3) Cathartic Therapy

(A) Psychoanalytic (B) Psychodrama (C) Primal Therapy

(4) Transactional Analysis

(5) Reality Therapy

(6) Cognitive Therapy

(A) Rational Emotive Therapy (B) Cognitive Skill Development

(7) Group Therapy

(A) Supportive (B) Confrontive

(8) Family Therapy

(9) Behavior Modification

(A) Reward-Punishment Contingencies (B) Aversive Conditioning

(C) Relaxation-Desensitization (D) Social Drinking Training

(10) Social Skills Training

(A) Assertive Training (B) Role Playing (C) Trial Situation

(11) Values Clarification

(12) Personal Power Development

(13) Educational (films, lectures, etc.)

(14) Self-Expression

(A) Poetry (B) Dance (C) Art (D) Music (E) Hobbies

(15) Community Reintegration

(A) Time Structuring (B) Community Planning (e.g., nonalcoholic nightclubs)

(16) Structured Environment

(A) Half-way House (B) Nursing/Boarding Home
(C) Total Community Setting

(17) Work Program – Vocational Training

(18) Inspirational – Meditation

(19) Antabuse

(20) Health Maintenance – Nutrition

(21) Chemotherapy (Tranquilizers, etc.)

(22) Milieu Therapy (Several of the above with no primary focus)

On the internet I discovered the websites of 28 addiction treatment centers from the Greater New Orleans area to the Greater Baton Rouge area. Nearly all of these treatment centers treated both alcohol and drug dependencies and had inpatient and outpatient program. Most had one or more psychological therapies. Sixteen (16) of these programs had a 12 Step program. Three (3) facilities were specifically religious based. Five (5) programs used drugs that target opioid receptors. Two (2) programs were based on brain restoration, one treatment facility used reality therapy, and another was based on Scientology.

Religions and meditation/mindfulness go back a few thousand years. Alcoholics Anonymous was created in the 1930's and is still the most popular treatment for addiction. Behavioral therapies and Scientology go back to the 1950's. Cognitive Behavior therapies go back to the 1960's. Methadone therapy was popular in the 1970's. The only thing "new" in the treatment of addictions is Motivational Interviewing which began in the 1990's. However, this method has a lot in common with non-directive therapy which began in the 1940's.

So how does the treatment of addictions line up with treating diabetes, hypertension and asthma? Has nothing new occurred within the last 40 years for these other illnesses?

Most of the above therapeutic methods used by addiction treatment programs have studies that support their effectiveness. I have several problems with these studies that support "evidence-based" treatment.

First of all, people are still doing studies that compare a treatment method with the control group having "no treatment". Pharmaceutical companies have long ago given up comparing a medicine against nothing. Double blind studies using a placebo in the control group is standard procedure. The power of a placebo is well known. Two placebos are better than one and a placebo that produces side effects is even better. A rule of thumb is that placebos do up to 30% better than no treatment. Consequently, if a treatment program is 20% better than a no treatment, you might only be measuring a placebo effect. In other words, I could have subjects stand on their heads for two hours per day to "clear the toxins" and do significantly better than the group waiting for treatment.

Of course, choosing a placebo treatment control group takes some creativity. The simplest placebo would be to offer the control group a medicine that they are told will reduce their cravings. An injection would probably work the best. Sham acupuncture or the use of mild electrical currents to alter one's "neuro receptors" would also be a good placebo.

Many treatment studies have compared one method against another instead of using a control group. Unfortunately, these studies usually conclude that both methods are equally successful, including a 27-million-dollar study on treating alcoholism conducted in 1997 (*BioMed Central*, 2005, 5(75)). However, without a true control group, the two methods might be equally unsuccessful. You have to have a control group, even if you are comparing two treatments against each other. I have my own idea for a control group that I will talk about later.

The second problem I have with evidence-based research is that the gains might be statistically significant but are rather small. The following example highlights this problem.

Cognitive Behavioral Therapy (CBT)

I found a meta-analysis of cognitive-behavioral treatment of drug abuse in a 2009 *Journal of Studies on Alcohol & Drugs*, Jul. 70(4). A meta-analysis means the researchers looked over a variety of similar studies for possible conclusions. Their conclusions are as follows:

"Across studies, CBT produced a **small** but statistically significant treatment effect (g = 0.154, p < .005). The pooled effect was somewhat lower at 6-9 months (g = 0.115, p < .005) and continued to diminish at 12-month follow-up (g = 0.096, p < .05). The effect of CBT was largest in marijuana studies (g = 0.513, p < .005) and in studies with a no-treatment control as the comparison condition (g = 0.796, p < .005). Meta-regression analyses indicated that the percentage of female participants was positively associated and the number of treatment sessions was negatively associated with effect size."

My first concern is what do they mean by "small"? If the median difference in relapse rates between the two groups was 12% (such as 68% vs 56%), anyone could understand this. It would mean that the treatment groups had 12% less relapses than the control groups.

You need the 'g' score and sample size to determine statistical significance. Achieving statistical significance is common when your sample sizes are very large. How many people can interpret a 'g' score of 0.154? A rule of thumb is that a 'g' score below .2 is small and a 'g' score above .8 is large. Note that the 'g' score drops 38% at a 12-month follow-up (.154-.096)/.154).

Second, clearly the studies with a no-treatment control group had by far the largest 'g' score (.796). In other words, had the researchers excluded those studies from their meta-analysis, the "small" treatment effect would have been "very small".

In summary, you need to study advanced statistics to understand a 'g' score. Anyone can understand relapse rates over time. Of course, you can publish both figures.

I am a big believer in cognitive therapy. I had the pleasure of talking to Albert Ellis, the founder of Rational Emotive Therapy. His simple but brilliant idea was that it is not what happens to us that is important but our <u>interpretation</u> of what happens to us that counts. If you were fired from a job you might attribute it to your boss being intimidated by your brilliance or that you are simply incompetent.

I have discovered that the application of Cognitive-Behavioral therapy tends to be a lot more cognitive than behavioral. The criterion for behavior therapy is a chart of behavior over time. There are over three dozen studies that say contingency management does better than treatments that do not use it (Stitzer & Petry, *Annual Review of Clinical Psychology*, 2006, 2). A review of over 30 studies found contingency management to increase the effectiveness of methadone treatment with outpatients (J.D. Griffith et al, *Drug and Alcohol Dependence*, 2000, 58). Reinforcement sessions for clean urine lasted from 12 to 18 weeks. Apparently, cash for drug-free urine or attending treatment sessions works best ($15 - $100). For additional information, *Reinforcement-Based Treatment for Substance Use Disorders,* (L. Michelle Tuton et al, American Psychological Association,2012), is an entire book dedicated to a behavioral approach to drug abuse.

One of the simplest behavioral techniques that anyone can use is to track your daily activities in a journal. Almost by definition, spending too much time at any one activity is an addiction. In addition to drug use – gambling, eating, sex and gaming can be addictions. Today, the average person spends about nine hours per day with an electronic device (i.e., television, cell phone, computer). Remember the phrase "workaholic"? Physicians often work fifty hours or more per week and are frequently stressed and die young. Our ancestors spent most of their time outdoors involved in physical activities. The least you can do is schedule periods of low stress-free time on a daily or weekly basis.

Treatment for addiction is going to require a variety of life style behavior changes that are not drug specific. Behaviorists all use something similar to the following "SMART" guidelines for setting behavioral goals.

- **S**pecific – clear and detailed
- **M**easurable – Something that can be charted
- **A**ttainable – Building on small steps
- **R**elevant – Will definitely improve your life
- **T**ime Bound – Realistic points in time to verify progress

You can set up your own reward system for meeting goals. When I worked with people trying to stop smoking, I had them place money in a jar for every cigarette not smoked that was less than their previous average. I also had them surround the jar with pictures and objects representing their goals and projected rewards including healthy smiling faces. A rule of thumb is that new behaviors need at least 10 weeks to become your new habits.

Alcoholic Anonymous/Narcotics Anonymous

I am not very familiar with Narcotics Anonymous (NA) so I am going to talk about Alcoholics Anonymous (AA). There are many studies on AA and the results are all over the map. There are studies that show it is great and studies that show it is ineffective. One study found a 48% abstinence at one year for those in AA versus a 24% abstinence rate for those without AA (Kaskutas, *Journal of Addictive Diseases*, 2009, 28(2)). The Cochrane Collaboration, founded in 1993, did a meta-analysis of eight studies in 2006 involving over 3000 individuals and found "no significant difference between the results of AA and twelve-step participation compared to other treatments".

I believe that the best thing about AA is having a sponsor. If you want to know what a sponsor does, watch the television program called "Mom". A sponsor can literally save your life. One study (*Psychological Addictive Behavior*, Sep. 2010) found that 42% of those with a sponsor were abstinent after one year versus 13% without a sponsor. Although this study did not control for motivation, it still shows one huge difference! Being a sponsor is just as good as having one. Another study found "Among those who were helping other alcoholics,

40% of participants avoided taking a drink in the year after treatment, whereas, among those who were not helping other alcoholics, only 22% avoided taking a drink" (*Journal of Studies on Alcoholism*, Nov. 2004). Having your spouse in AL Anon also helps the person in AA recover.

While giving a lecture on addiction, I was told that if I was not a recovering alcoholic, I was not fit to give advice about alcoholism. My response was "I cannot say what it is like to be an alcoholic. On the other hand, if you are not a statistician, you cannot tell me what works and what doesn't. Here is my hypothetical example.

It occurred to me that if an alcoholic could only reach for a book instead of a drink, this might lead to a cure. The more often a person uses this response when having an urge to drink, the more effective it will become. Once absorbed in a book, one's craving for alcohol will diminish.

To sustain this effect, I will create a "Book Club for Alcoholics". Once a week, they can meet to discuss the latest book they are reading. Members of this book club will reinforce each other's behavior to maintain abstinence while at the same time benefiting from the enjoyment and learning of reading.

Suppose I created this new therapy and treated alcoholics for several months. Six months later I visited a "Book Club for Alcoholics". To my amazement they were all happy and doing well. One of the ten members told me how this book club saved his life. Another member told me how nothing worked for her until she joined this club.

A third member told of having a relapse but with the support of the group regained his sobriety. I thought to myself, I am a genius!

Then it occurred to me that I had dealt with fifty people during the early months of my treatment. What became of the other forty people? So, I tracked them down six months after treatment and discovered the following:

(A) Twenty-four (24) persons never attended the book club. Of those 24, 15 had relapsed and 8 were sober and 1 had died.
(B) Sixteen (16) others attended the book club but eventually dropped out. Of those 16, 10 had relapsed and 6 were sober.
(C) I had already discovered that of the 10 who were still in the book club, 9 were sober and one relapsed.

Consequently, my book club therapy for alcoholics led to 23 remaining sober for six months with 26 relapsing and 1 undetermined death. In other words, my success rate for six months was 23/49 or 47%. Evidently, I am not a genius after all, although my success rate is on par with other treatment programs.

However, there would be people in my "Book Club for Alcoholics" who would swear by it as THE treatment for alcoholics. Unfortunately, they are not statisticians!

Note: There are other addiction recovery groups such as SMART Recovery and Secular Organizations for Sobriety. There is even Moderation Management for problem drinkers. A lot of recovery groups have sprung up to help persons with drug abuse. Most of these groups were conceived by former users. According to Ryan Hampton (*American Fix*), The Facing Addiction Action Network has over 600 groups to help people recover. The best thing about these groups is that they are <u>free</u>. Certainly, former addicts know things that people who do research do not know and vice-versa.

I believe, that in general, if something is powerful enough to help you, it also has the potential for hurting you. Suppose a pharmaceutical company developed a drug that when they first tried it out on a sample of 20 people, 10 of those people showed marked improvements. If the pharmaceutical industry did not have any regulations, they would immediately market this drug to the masses. They might discover that although it leads to definite improvement in 50% of the people who take it, 2% die from it. Would you take this drug? There is no question that it helps a lot more people than it harms. Perhaps this new drug works but you need to keep taking it to stay well. Unfortunately, long-term use of this drug produces Parkinson like symptoms. Would you still take it?

Of course, medications differ from support groups. I am a big believer in support groups. Still, they are not without potential problems. Suppose Alcoholics Anonymous (AA) helps a man stop drinking. Two years later he is celebrating a wedding with friends and he takes a drink. Is it possible that his subconscious tells him that "you can only refuse the first drink"? This is what AA says. Therefore, he feels compelled to take another drink.

Self-help groups need research as much paid treatment groups do. Pre and post testing with control groups over time and space (geography) is the only way I know of to verify a group's effectiveness. Testimonials don't cut it. Perhaps the charisma of the group's founder is what makes it work initially. Perhaps most of the gains represent the placebo effect or the attention of sympathetic people. Selective attention allows people to focus on the prominent successes while ignoring the people who slip away to continue their drug use. Even psychology with its Ph.D.'s has fads. What became of primal therapy and transactional analysis?

AA teaches that you are an alcoholic for life. The best you can be is a recovering alcoholic. A 1976 Rand Corporation study of over 2,000 men from 44 different treatment centers reported 22% of the men were drinking moderately 18 months after treatment. I did an anonymous study of 190 patients at four Minnesota state hospitals. 19% of those intended to control or moderate their drinking even though all of the hospitals taught abstinence.

Medication Assisted Therapy (MAT)

Most experts on drug abuse recommend the use of drugs to take up opioid receptors (agonists) or block opioid receptors (antagonists) to supplement standard treatment. A study was done "at eight US community-based inpatient services conducted between 2014 and 2016 to test their effectiveness. It placed about half of its 570 participants into naltrexone treatment (antagonist), and the other half into buprenorphine treatment (agonist). Then it tracked their relapse rates over 24 weeks (about half a year)." The study found the opioid relapse rate was about 52 percent for naltrexone. For buprenorphine, it was 56 percent (Sponsored by the NIDA and published in *The Lancet* in 2017).

Although methadone was available in the 1970's, buprenorphine is safer to use and was not officially approved to treat opioid addiction until 2002. Some people believe you can go from methadone to buprenorphine to naltrexone.

Several sources believe the use of opioid antagonists are underutilized in the United States. Physicians need eight hours of training to prescribe buprenorphine. Less than 5% are thus certified. Only 5 of my 26 treatment center websites mentioned the use of one or more of these drugs. Europe and Scandinavia are more likely to use this type of drug. In fact, Finland uses an opioid antagonist called nalmefene which is seldom used here even though an injectable form of the drug was approved in the United States in 1995 as an antidote for opioid overdose.

According to an article in *Scientific American Mind*, Mar/Apr, 2013:

- Drug use impairs the brain's flexibility, making it difficult to change habits.

- Neural communication is impaired by broken machinery at the synapses – the connections between brain cells.
- Repairing this machinery with pharmacological treatment can restore flexibility, allowing an addict's desire to change to triumph over his or her habit.

The most common medications for the addictions are as follows:

Opioid Addiction: Methadone, Naltrexone, Buprenorphine, Naloxone

Alcohol Addiction: Acamprosate, Naltrexone, Disulfiram, Ondansetron
(Ondansetron reduces cravings in early onset drinkers.)

Tobacco/Nicotine Addiction: Bupropion, Varenicline

Cocaine Addiction: Modafinil, Disulfiram

Methamphetamine Addiction: None (One in the works - ibudilast)

N-benzylpiperazine (BZP) has similarities to Methamphetamine. New Zealand is experimenting with this drug as a replacement therapy. It is an illegal drug in the United States.

Each drug (abused drug and medication) has its own unique properties. An advantage Methadone has over Heroin is that is lasts for a day instead of a few hours. Unfortunately, many addicts abuse more than one drug.

Methadone and alcohol can be a deadly combination. So can Methadone with a benzodiazepine (e.g., Valium, Librium, Xanax). Buprenorphine is safer than Methadone because it is absorbed under the tongue making an overdose rare. Some medicines like Suboxone are a combination of the above (Buprenorphine and Naloxone). A complete review of how opioid medicines work and how to use them can be found in *"Overcoming Opioid Addiction"* by Adam Bisaga.

In the case of alcohol addiction, naltrexone is an antagonist blocking opioid receptors and possibly reducing the rewarding effects of alcohol. Acamprosate affects the production of glutamate. Ondansetron reduces the activity of a serotonin receptor.

We have made gains in discovering the neurological pathways of addiction. A medication to use up or block the receptors of opioids is a good idea. However, fifty years ago we had Antabuse (Disulfiram) to discourage the consumption of alcohol. Of course, it only works if the patient continues to take it daily. Vivitrol (Naltrexone) by injection works for a month. Buprenorphine can now be given as a monthly injection (Sublocade) or even with an implant that lasts for six months (Probuphine). Alcoholics Anonymous discouraged the use of Antabuse in my day. Even today, some people still do not like the idea of treating drug addiction with a drug.

Family Therapy

Guess what? I have a fourth problem with evidenced-based treatment. I know what contingency management is. I have a pretty good idea of what cognitive therapy is. I don't know what specific criteria must be met to be called family therapy. This is embarrassing because I've done family therapy. As best as I remember, what I did depended on the family.

For example, I might work with one family that is fairly intact. They can express their caring and support for the family member addicted to drugs. They can also set rules that provide for consequences to the addict's behaviors. They can appropriately reward "good" behaviors and provide sanctions for "bad" behaviors. They can make an effort to reintegrate the addict into the normal day to day affairs of the family. With this family, we have a good chance of success with helping this addict recover.

On the other hand, I may have a dysfunctional family where everyone has their own problems. The father might be cold and punitive. The mother might easily cave in to inadvertently supporting the addict's habit (i.e., an enabler). A sister may have tuned out everyone in the family to go her own way. A brother may feel jealous of all of the attention given to the addict. In this case, my chances of success with helping this person recover from his addiction with family therapy is small.

So how can you accurately measure something that changes from family to family? I might have had great success with one family and next to nothing on another family. I read that multidimensional family therapy is even better than traditional family therapy. Good luck on finding an operational measure for that.

Community Reinforcement and Family Therapy (CRAFT) was created specifically for families of addicts. CRAFT teaches families how to interact with an addict without using detachment or confrontation. This approach apparently works well with the mothers of adult children. Note that a Community Reinforcement Approach (CRA) was used for alcoholism in the late 1970's.

M. Duncan Stanton and others did a meta-analysis of family/couple's therapy that a statistician could love (*Psychological Bulletin*, 1997, 122(2)). They reviewed 15 studies with each study having many couples (Total N = 1,571). They only looked at studies that had at least two comparisons, subjects were randomly assigned, and follow-up was at least a year or more. They even did their best to account for dropouts. Whereas there was a lot of variation between studies, overall results indicated that family therapy was better than individual counseling or peer group therapy. One study with juvenile offenders found that individual counseling led to more than four times the arrests over a four-year period than those who received family therapy.

The research clearly supports family therapy. However, any support a substance abuser receives from significant others will reduce his chances of recidivism. Of course, family therapy is not recommended for addiction treatment when the family is clearly a hostile environment or when domestic violence is involved. In these cases, it is best to wait until the client has favorably stabilized.

Counseling

Even if I were to visit the local treatment centers for addiction, I could not make a recommendation. Why? Because I believe the most important part of treatment is the person's individual counselor. Even if this person is mostly a coordinator of various activities, he or she is probably instrumental in setting the client's expectations and providing comfort and guidance when necessary. Many books on addiction recommend a certified counselor. Some counselors have specialties. Is your counselor as good as the ones who do research in that specialty? A. Thomas McLellan says "There are no published studies validating whether patients treated by "certified" addictions counselors, physicians, or psychologists have better outcomes than patients treated by noncertified individuals" (*Rethinking Substance Abuse*, Miller et al, 2006, p. 282).

If the states really believed in evidenced-based treatment, they would not require counselors to have advanced degrees. This is not because we are lacking evidence. In fact, over 30 studies show that persons with advanced degrees are <u>not</u> the best counselors. It is all in my book "*Counseling: A Profession or a Trade?*" (Chapter 9, Amazon). These studies were done in the 1980's and quickly forgotten (i.e., not available on the Internet). Furthermore, to the best of my knowledge, there is not a single study that compares people who score high on the licensure tests with counseling success. This is another fiction of what a psychologist would call "face validity". I play the trumpet. I like to say that with a music degree and a multiple-choice test, I could be playing with a major symphony orchestra. Unfortunately, they would probably insist on hearing me play the trumpet first.

One of the biggest problems with choosing a counselor with an advanced degree is that few colleges truly screen people wanting to be counselors. If you have a 4.0 grade point average, you can get admission to over 90% of the counseling programs being offered. Books on counseling all believe the following characteristics make good counselors – empathy and compassion, nonjudgmental, and being a good listener. Guess what? Few counseling programs, if any, screen people for these qualities to gain admission. I have 96 semester credit hours in psychology. I have never seen a course titled "Developing Empathy". Why? Because if you are not an empathetic and compassionate person by the time you are 21, you are not likely to become one. The same is true for the other two characteristics. When I ran a program for chemical dependency, I hired a person with all of the above characteristics to be the counselor. He had a bachelor's degree in recreation!

According to William R. Miller, the following methods are effective for counseling for alcoholism (Taken directly from *Rethinking Substance Abuse*):

1) Feedback regarding personal status, relative to norms, of drinking and its consequences.

2) Responsibility for change is left with the client, honoring the person's autonomy.
3) Advice and encouragement to reduce or stop drinking.
4) Menu of options for how to change one's drinking.
5) Empathic counseling style that listens to the client.
6) Support for self-efficacy, and optimism about the possibilities for change.

Just as I believe in behavior checklists for clients, I believe in behavior checklist for counselors. Counselors could be videotaped over several sessions to observe how they actually behave with a client. I would not be surprised if counselors varied from one another more on dimensions such as:

1) The ratio of counselor talking to client talking
2) The number of times they offer encouragement
3) The amount of advice they give
4) The amount of homework they give

than on their use of cognitive, behavioral, motivational interviewing and other techniques. Similar to my advice on getting rid of diagnostic labels based on logic and theory, we could eventually discover the real types of counselors based on behavior clusters using a modified factor analysis. Do you really believe that Cognitive-Behavioral counselors are alike?

I created many surveys when I evaluated educational programs for three years. Tests and surveys need the assistance of a qualified statistician. Items chosen need to be reliable, valid, specific and necessary.

My Counselor Survey (Appendix 5) is a prototype. Interviews with clients might lead you to discover that people differ on their interpretation of "homework" (Item 5). You might also discover than the ratings on "knowledgeable" (item 13) and "helpful" (item 14) are highly correlated. You would then need to either drop one of the questions, rewrite the questions, or combine the questions. Most surveys suffer from a halo effect (e.g., high intercorrelations of items). I prefer forced-choice surveys and rank ordering. Knowing people want a wall tells you something. Knowing they would prefer a wall over paying down the federal deficit tells you more. Having people show their preferences by rank ordering ten ways the government could spend its money tells you a lot. Republicans and Democrats might differ on the top three priorities but agree on their fourth choice. That would be valuable information. Furthermore, every survey should allow for write-in comments, even if a computer cannot process them.

Motivational Interviewing

This brings us to "motivational interviewing". Psychologists believe that a label makes something real. As best as I can tell, a good counselor has always done motivational interviewing. In other words, you listen to the voice of the counselor. In Statistical Process Control, used to improve manufacturing, you listen to the voice of the process. From listening to the client, you can determine where he is presently at, where he wants to be, what he thinks he needs to do to get there, and why he hasn't already done this on his own.

Before you believe motivational interviewing is new, read about non-directive counseling. Non-directive counseling began in the 1940's with Carl Rogers. According the American Psychological Association Dictionary, nondirective counseling is "an orderly process of client self-discovery and actualization that occurs in response to the therapist's consistent empathic understanding of, acceptance of, and respect for the client's frame. The therapist sets the stage for personality growth by reflecting and clarifying the ideas of the client, who is able to see himself or herself more clearly and come into closer touch with his or her real self. As therapy progresses, the client resolves conflicts, reorganizes values and approaches to life, and learns how to interpret his or her thoughts and feelings, consequently changing behavior that he or she considers problematic."

With motivational interviewing (MI), the counselor decides what stage the client is in and how to help move him to the next stage. This new idea forms the basis of MI. The stages of change include:

1. Precontemplation
2. Contemplation
3. Preparation
4. Action
5. Maintenance

A counselor is not like an auto mechanic. An auto mechanic does not care about your opinion when all of his tests indicate your car needs a new transmission. Ironically, knowing too much about addiction can create as many problems as it solves. When I worked with alcoholics, it was my opinion that former alcoholics made both the best and the worst counselors. The best counselors were compassionate and persistent. The worst counselors thought that what worked for them should work for everybody.

Sometimes knowing too much gets in the way. I ran a data processing office for several years. I had two people under me with master's degrees in computer science. They certainly knew more about data processing than I did. However, my boss wanted a people person (compared with ADP personalities) in charge who could balance the ideas of others. Managing and counseling are specialties in themselves. Perhaps it is best that an addiction counselor knows about counseling rather than about addiction.

One of the trickiest things about counseling is giving advice. This is why the medical model does not work well for counselors. Physicians give a patient advice and then blame the patient when he or she doesn't follow it. They rely on their authority to get things done and this often works for them. Unfortunately, a counselor who gives good advice has taught the client that he needs to rely on others. One the other hand, a counselor who gives bad advice will discourage a person from seeking help when he needs it. In other words, good counselors should be facilitators, not givers of advice. They may present information and discuss possibilities but always let the client make the decisions. If you want a quick view on what I believe makes a good counselor, see "Choosing a Counselor – What others will not tell you" on YouTube.

Do you really believe that physicians trained in drug abuse are not going to recommend using an agonist like buprenorphine or an antagonist like naltrexone? Will they simply discuss its use and leave the choice up to the client? If the client makes what turns out to be a bad choice, will he learn something? Of course, the powers that be have to be authoritative when the decision is a life or death one. We commit people when necessary and give them naloxone to save their lives.

If you are a Ph.D. psychologist and believe in Motivational Interviewing, the first thing you should do is give up the "doctor" title. It doesn't matter what you think; most people are going to respond to the doctor title as if you are an authority. Consequently, they are going to ask for and expect advice. (I just excluded a few thousand people from claiming they are disciples of Motivational Interviewing.) A good compromise is to allow a Ph.D. or an M.D. after your name while dropping the title.

Am I a hypocrite? Isn't this whole book full of advice? Yes and no. I do not know you personally so consider what I say as "suggestions" that may or may not apply to you. Likewise, I am not familiar with what every state is doing for drug addiction nor do I know what is happening at the National Institute of Drug Abuse. And yes, I went by the doctor title at Brainerd State Hospital when I was young and naïve. I actually believe that even physicians should give up the doctor title. The reasons are in my Amazon book *"Merit – The Forgotten Dimension in Choosing an Occupation"*.

Brief Intervention

Although brief intervention isn't exactly a type of treatment, it deserves special mention because there are several studies that show how powerful this can be. The power of brief intervention is less surprising when you realize that most people who recover from drug problems do so on their own. A review of brief intervention (1 to 3 sessions) for alcohol abuse led to a 24% reduction in alcohol consumption (A. Moyer et al, *Addiction*, 2002, 97(3)). Not surprisingly, brief intervention does not work well with the most serious cases. (Statistical Note: Comparing brief treatment with long-term treatment to see if they are equally effective would be trying to prove the null hypothesis. In other words, you can only test if one method is better than another.)

Brief intervention avoids the stigma of labeling someone as an addict. Furthermore, brief intervention completely avoids the concept of needing to "hit bottom". Not everyone wants to see themselves as having a chronic illness. Failure at self-change is considered to be one of the defining characteristics of dependency. Brief intervention can be particularly effective with a person who is already in the contemplative stage and needs that extra push into preparation and action. Having commitment and a plan are the best predictors of improvement. Some people believe that everyone has a "tipping point" where progress accelerates. A rule of thumb in Motivational Interviewing and Nondirective counseling is that a person is more likely to follow though with his own idea than an idea created by someone else. If you are old enough to remember the television character Sgt. Bilko, you know he was famous for convincing others that his ideas were really theirs. Perhaps honesty is not always the best counseling technique.

Individual Treatment

My specialty in psychology was individual differences. Not surprisingly, I categorized alcoholics into eight different types, the goals for each type and the primary and secondary means to achieve them. For each of the types, I created a learning path with motive, situation, response and initial and delayed consequences (see Appendix 1). Many of the books that I have read about addiction believe there is a solution. I disagree. I believe there are solutions.

Cognitive therapy is great for people with distorted beliefs. These include people who are depressed, anxious, perfectionists, narcissists, paranoid, and people who think that their political party is always right. On the other hand, if you take drugs because your friends take drugs, you need new friends, not new beliefs.

The definition of maturity is delaying immediate gratification for long-term gratification. You can study hard, get a job and work hard and eventually have enough money to buy a boat and go to Disneyworld with the family; or you can feel good right now with drugs.

Unfortunately, treatment centers are faced with the fact that drug users and alcoholics all look pretty much alike when they reach the bottom (i.e., no job, no spouse, poor health). However, there are:

(1) People who started on drugs because of their peers
(2) People who took drugs to overcome depression, anxiety or even schizophrenia, and
(3) People who thought that going to school, getting a job and working hard was too long a wait for the good life or thought that their life would be short after seeing friends die in turf wars.

Each of these people need a different treatment approach. The second group is stressed and often over-socialized and could benefit from cognitive therapy. The third group is usually immature and under socialized and could benefit from AA or NA. The first group needs a cultural approach that I will discuss later.

Ironically, the 40-year-old man whose wife divorced him, then got "high", and then lost his job might come to treatment looking worse than the 20-year-old who is unemployed and living at home with his parents. Nevertheless, the 40-year-old might quickly recover with traditional Cognitive-Behavioral therapy. On the other hand, how long will it take for the 20-year-old to go from the maturity of a 14-year-old, the age when he first started on drugs, to an adult?

Even if you think my three types are somewhat trivial, you should at least determine when an addict first began using. A rule of thumb is – the earlier drug abuse started, the longer the treatment needed. We already know that the probability of becoming addicted decreases for those starting drugs at a later age (Roughly 50% at 14, 9% after 22) although this varies with the drug used.

The Center for Prisoner Health and Human Rights says that approximately half of prison and jail inmates meet DSM-IV criteria for substance abuse or dependence. How should this population be treated? Note that very few prisons use medication-assisted treatment. Women on drugs who are pregnant are another special case of addicts. We have separate treatment centers for adolescents and women. What about LGBT persons? What about the elderly? People tend to be more comfortable with others like themselves, even if the treatment methods are the same.

There exists very little research on treating teenagers who abuse drugs. Do they require inpatient treatment and should the inpatient treatment specialize in teenagers? Are they good candidates for Medication-Assisted treatment? How should the parents be involved? Do school prevention programs help? We know that not even alcohol or marijuana are good for the developing brain, let alone opioids and other street drugs.

My answer is the same. More individual studies are needed, but there is no substitute for a state system that does both diagnosis, referral and follow-up to see what works for whom in the everyday world. Of course, we will always need research. Research studies rely on randomly assigning subjects to different groups. Research studies can employ a variety of pre and post measures relevant to the hypothesis being tested. Eventually, what research finds promising needs to be incorporated into everyday therapy. It would be naive to think that the results will be the same. Additional verification is needed.

One of the most important decisions a potential client needs to make is "where to go for treatment?". When is the last time you saw a research article that compared different treatment centers as opposed to different treatment methods? As pointed out by Ryan Hampton in *American Fix* (2018), addiction treatment centers **pay** people to find them clients. Presently, I do not believe there is a good way for choosing an addiction treatment center. As I point out in "Choosing a Counselor – What others will not tell you" (YouTube), you cannot find a good counselor by asking the right questions. You can only determine if your counselor is good after being in treatment for several sessions.

The best research projects do more than show how effective a treatment procedure is, they show how effective it is for whom. This is a third problem with evidence-based programs. An evidence-based therapy might help 60% or the clients while 40% of the clients are not being helped because they are in the wrong type of therapy for them. This may explain, in part, the small gains mentioned earlier for Cognitive-Behavior therapy. Not surprisingly, clients are less likely to drop out of a treatment they preferred (Lindhiem et al, *Clinical Psychology Review*, August, 2014).

Not enough research looks at how therapy relates to individual differences. Today the big five are extraversion, neuroticism, conscientiousness, agreeableness, and openness. I always like the 16 types of personality based on extraversion vs introversion, intuition vs sensation, thinking vs feeling and judging vs perceiving (Myers-Briggs). Surprisingly, I cannot find a study that tests whether introverts do better with individual therapy whereas extroverts do better with group therapy. I would think that persons who score high on the "Psychopathic" MMPI scale need a group (peer pressure) and a sponsor. Drug users who are anti-social with the most problems controlling their behaviors tend to have the worse prognoses. Unfortunately, most of these persons end up in our correctional system where treatment options are limited. Person with co-occurring psychiatric disorders also have a poor prognosis and need special assistance.

Those people who score high on the Neuroticism scale probably need Cognitive therapy. Not surprisingly, male addicts are more likely to be anti-social while females are more likely to be anxious and depressed. I would expect that persons who are "Conscientious" would be most likely to stick with a program. I have my own idea of a specific treatment for those addicts who are sensation seekers that I will discuss under "New Approaches to Drug Addiction".

Given that the courts refer a lot of males to addiction treatment and that the prognosis for persons with conduct disorders is not good, it makes sense that we should have addiction treatment centers that specialize in this population. Outward bound type programs might be well suited for these people. One thing administrators must realize is that <u>punishment is an attitude</u>. Some of the early treatment centers for drug addiction used demeaning activities for newcomers like using a toothbrush to clean something. One the other hand, I have never met a former Marine who complained about being inappropriately punished. Carrying a heavy backpack for miles is training, not punishment.

I believe a “bootcamp” approach to drug addiction treatment for antisocial personalities needs the following four attitudes. One, you are stronger than you realize. Two, our training will give you skills you can use later. Three, what you learn here may save your life someday. Four, there are times you have to rely on others and they have to rely on you. I have a friend who took survival skills for northern Minnesota in the winter. He had to fall through the ice and stay alive! Perhaps once you realize how tough you can be, saying “no” to drugs isn’t so hard.

Many treatment centers talk about treating the whole person. You might like a wholistic family physician. Suppose you got cancer. Do you stick with your doctor who treats the whole person or do you go to a cancer specialist? Are there presently treatment specialists in drug addiction? NA is a specialty. So is a nutritional approach. Giving out opioid agonists such as buprenorphine or suboxone is also a specialty.

Unfortunately, I know of no addiction specialties based on personality.

Researchers from the University of Pennsylvania discovered that the epilepsy drug topiramate helped heavy drinkers cut back but only if they had a particular gene found in people of European descent (*Times Picayune*, Jan. 2, 2015). Expect more treatments in the future to differ based on a person's biology/genetics.

Addiction treatment centers are the enemy of individual differences and it is not their fault. Addiction treatment centers are in the business of making money. They do not like turning people away. Do you think they have ever told someone "You are a shy introvert. You would be better off with an individual counselor"? Do you think they have ever said "We do not have much experience with someone addicted to Ayahuasca or sniffing glue or diet pills or steroids? Every treatment center claims they offer individual treatment. Therefore, you should ask what tests they administer and what questions they ask to determine a person's individuality. Then ask for examples of how people are treated differently.

Furthermore, pharmaceutical companies do not like to measure individual differences. There is a lot more money in claiming a remedy for arthritis if it applies to all types of arthritis and all types of people.

Medicine is full of specialties and even your primary physician might refer you to a specialist. Of course, physicians are often overbooked. They do not need your business. As previously mentioned, no one who does diagnosis and referral should be in the addiction treatment business. It is a conflict of interests.

I believe that treatment centers need a separate program for readmissions. Nobody likes to repeat the third grade. Readmissions seldom need to recognize that they really do have a problem. How much can be learned by repeating the twelve steps? This is an area where individualized treatment really counts. What led up to a relapse? Was it stress? An unrecognized cue? Peer pressure? Negative thinking? No one to intervene? No job? Readmission does not imply nothing was successful in the first treatment. Each effort "primes the pump". The fact that you get water after the fifth prime does not imply that the first four were of no value.

Another possible group that needs special treatment are binge users. Binge drinkers are the most likely to die from alcohol poisoning. According to the Center for Disease Control, three out of four people who die from binge drinking are between the ages of 35 and 65 (*Times Picayune*, Jan. 7, 2015). Guess what? Many of these people are not even considered to be addicted!

Do individual differences determine your drug of choice? Maia Szalavitz in *Unbroken Brain* mentions the possibility that cocaine users seek excitement whereas opioid users want to feel comfortable. She thinks cocaine use might be associated with "wanting" whereas opioid use is associated with "liking". She believes that "wanting" is more powerful than "liking". Although I claim individual differences as my specialty, I know very little about why people choose the drug they do. A rule of thumb is that seeking pleasure is related to impulse disorders and relief of anxiety is related to compulsive disorders.

Of course, it is not unusual for an addict to use more than one drug. Even recovering alcoholics tend to be big smokers and coffee drinkers. One possibility is that addicts have learned to associate drugs with quick pleasure. This would be true of people who are immature and by definition do not like to postpone immediate gratification for long term gains.

To my knowledge there are few studies that show the value of matching personalities to type of treatment. Even that 27-million-dollar study comparing different treatments for alcoholics could not find any striking differences. In other words, I believe the major effects of any treatment program is keeping people sober/clean for 30 or more days with the expectation of living a life without addicting drugs. I present my own example of an addiction control group later that will measure this effect. Additional gains from actual treatment procedures are probably small. Adding the best match of personality and treatment can be expected to be even smaller. Keep in mind that a bad match of personality and treatment (an anxious introvert and group therapy?) might even be contraindicated.

There is one area where individual differences are critical to the type of counseling given drug addicts. For lack of a better word, we could call this “readiness for change”. This concept forms the basis of Motivational Interviewing.

Nearly everyone believes that genetics are important for drug abuse. One researcher estimates that addiction vulnerability has a 50% genetic basis (J.C. Wang et al, *Annual Review of Genomics in Human Genetics*, 2012, 13). According to Judith Grisel, "People's individual differences in a drug's rewarding effects, as well as the development of tolerance or dependence, have been associated with structural differences in the GABA(A) receptor (*Never Enough*, p. 112). Surprisingly, few research studies see if persons with a family history of addiction vary from the others on whatever measure they are testing.

Several sources comment on how minimal individual differences play in treating drug abuse. It is my opinion that the lack of evidence on the effect of individual differences on drug abuse treatment reflects how little we know about treating addicts. Presently, a lot of medical procedures treat everyone alike. That will change dramatically with the knowledge of genomes. Your medical file might also describe your microbiome (gut bacteria). At the same time, I predict that when genomes become popular in medicine, physicians will under-value the role of social history.

This brings us back to my main theme of the states moving away from treatment to do pre-evaluations and post-evaluations. Treating addiction presently has a 50% chance of succeeding. Gathering pre and post treatment data will allow us to maximize treatment by not only knowing which treatment centers are the most successful but in gathering data as to what works best for whom.

Populations and Samples

The discussion I am having here should be part of every book on addiction. I am following the section on individual differences for reasons that will become obvious.

The book "*Overcoming Opioid Addiction*" refers to the many studies that support medication-assisted treatment. If you are an elderly single Asian woman who lives in Hawaii who got hooked on heroin following a prescription, does this apply to you? It depends. How many of those studies included elderly single Asian women from Hawaii?

Rule 1: If you want to generalize to a population, the samples in your study must be representative of that population.

For starters, even though there are international journals on addiction, let us assume we are only interested in the United States. Here are some of the variables to consider if you want a study to be valid for the entire country:

1. You need to determine what is your population. Are they opioid drug abusers? All illegal drug users? Adolescent drug abusers?
2. All regions of the country need to be in your sample.
3. If 22% of addicts are women, how many women are in your sample?
4. Other segments of the population could also be represented proportionately which could

include Blacks, Hispanics, Asians, and Native Americans.

5. Socioeconomic data and level of education should be considered in your sample.
6. Percent of drug abusers with co-occurring disorders need to be considered.
7. Person involved with corrections need to be represented.

Rule 2: Using a sample that contains the same proportions of important categories as the general population is referred to as a "stratified sample". If your sample size is very large, you might be able to use a random sample by pulling from the entire population.

Rule 3: Consider doing studies with only special subpopulations. For example, you might want to study Hispanics only or a comparison of Hispanics, Blacks, and Caucasians. Another possibility would be to study only persons who became addicted to opioids from a prescription or only those addicts who end up in the correctional system.

Rule 4: Just as there are subgroups of subjects, there are various treatments. For example, you might want to see if the effectiveness of family therapy varies according to the socio-economic status of the subjects.

Rule 5: In addition to the interaction of subjects and treatments, there are different measures of change to consider as well as when to measure these changes.

Rule 6: A large sample size increases the probability that you will find significant differences. That is why you always need a measure of the strength for those differences.

If you think I am about to say this is another reason for distrusting "evidence-based" treatment, you would be wrong. Most studies describe the population of subjects involved. The problem is that book authors, such as myself, often present general findings and leave out the details. For example, I might say that several studies show that therapy 'X' is effective. What I might forget to mention is that these several studies involve only 58 people of which over 70% of the subjects are white single males. Consequently, 'X' therapy might have little value for married people, women, minorities or the elderly. If you take the time to thoroughly comb through the details of research studies, you might discover more information on individual differences than is typically reported.

The National Institute of Drug Abuse says that the relapse rates after treatment range from 40% to 60%. My guess is that 20% to 80% is more accurate. If you began drugs at an early age, live in a poor neighborhood, have no job skills, hobbies or friends, your chance of a relapse is probably close to 80%. If you are middle class with a job and family and did not get hooked until you took opioids for a back problem, your chance of relapsing is probably only about 20%, especially if your job is on the line. Insurance companies use actuaries (statisticians) to compute accident rates. They cannot make money with ballpark figures. We need to collect a lot more data on relapse rates for different people and situations. As mentioned previously, in the future each person will receive his or her own likelihood of relapsing in a year given one's biology, personality, history and treatment program.

One way to find individual differences is to look for "outliers". Most characteristics follow a normal bell-shaped curve. When several independent factors contribute to a characteristic being measured, the outcome is almost always a normal bell-shaped curve. Outliers usually represent too many subjects at one end of the curve. People who do cognitive therapy would probably tell me that so many studies have been done, it has been proven to be effective for everybody. My first response would be "point me to a study that uses cognitive therapy for persons with low I.Q.'s." I have worked with the developmentally disabled and have discovered that contingency management works far better with this population than cognitive therapy.

Another problem with finding individual differences is that you need large samples to show small differences. The way around this problem is to select only the type of people you are interested in studying and hopefully have a hypothesis on how they differ from most people with substance abuse.

When it comes to getting a representative sampling of the population, who could do a better job – research universities or state governments? Who is most likely to sample rural areas? Who has the easiest access to prisons? Who has a list of persons receiving public aid? Who can best chase down people who have moved to a different location in the state? Who is most likely to know that a former client of an addiction treatment center is presently receiving services elsewhere? Who has an ongoing budget for follow-up? It has been a known fact for years, that what we call psychology is mostly the psychology of university students.

New Approaches to Drug Addiction

Mindfulness

Although mindfulness is not really new, it has become popular over the last several years. Mindfulness actually dates back a few thousand years to a type of meditation/yoga. Mindfulness is focusing on being aware of what you're sensing and feeling in the moment without interpretation or judgment. It may also involve some basic breathing methods associated with hatha yoga.

The practice of mindfulness includes:

(1) Paying attention to the moment. Be aware of all of your senses – sights, sounds, body sensations such as touching, smells and tastes.

(2) Observe what is happening without judgment.

(3) Letting thoughts and sensations happen without trying to control where they are going including letting negative thoughts and feelings flow through you.

(4) Accepting yourself and your experiences.

(5) Focusing on your breathing and posture to be in a relaxed state. Sometimes gentle music helps.

Mindfulness will help you avoid the automatic triggers (classical conditioning) that are often associated with addictive behaviors. Have you ever driven to work without remembering what you saw along the way? Have you ever mindlessly eaten snacks while watching television? Mindfulness is the opposite of doing things automatically. Consequently, it seems well suited for addictions. Addictions involve letting conditioned physical urges dominate your life. With mindfulness, you acknowledge the urges and let them pass.

Mindfulness is particularly useful as a method of stress reduction. Meditation is one of the first cognitive therapies. There is considerable evidence that meditation reduces stress and anxiety based on psychological and physical measures. According to Garland and Howard in *Addiction Science Clinical Practice* (April, 2018) "These mindful qualities may serve as antidotes to addictive behavior; indeed, trait mindfulness, which has been correlated with enhanced cognitive control capacities [study reference], is significantly inversely associated with substance use [study reference] and craving [study reference], and positively associated with the ability to disengage attention and recover autonomic function following exposure to addiction-related cues [study references]".

Biological and Genetic Approaches

We know a lot about the biological foundations of addiction. Certain drugs cause a surge of dopamine, a neurotransmitter, in the nucleus accumbens. Dopamine can bind to 5 different receptors but D2 seems to be implicated for the addictive drugs. We know that some people (15%?) are genetically prone to addiction. These people tend to have a reward insufficiency. In other words, they seem to get fewer rewards from normal activities. However, certain drugs give them a "high" that most other people do not get. Furthermore, some people find the "high" from drugs to be overwhelming and therefore <u>not</u> rewarding.

Twin studies suggest that 40% to 60% of being prone to addiction is genetic. Environmental factors that increase the chances of addiction include stress and peer pressure. Increased tolerance to a drug means that a person needs to up the dose to get the same effects as before. Severe withdrawal symptoms can encourage a person to continue using.

Studies on rats given drugs discovered that the receptors that detect glutamate in the synapses begin to malfunction. Treating them with N-acetylcysteine (NAC) returned glutamate levels to normal (*Scientific Mind*, 2013,

Mar/Apr). Preliminary work with humans yielded modest results.

One study found that cortisol lead to reduced craving in low-dose heroin addicts (*Translational Psychiatry*, 2015, V5).

Creating vaccines to prevent addiction is currently in progress. Vaccines produce antibodies to keep a drug from entering the brain. A cocaine vaccine was tried out in 2009. According to an article in *Newsweek* (Mar. 15, 2010), "Only 38 percent of the coke users produced enough antibodies to dull the effects of cocaine, and, of those, only half stayed clean more than half the time."

It is possible that we may soon have an effective vaccine to prevent opioid addiction. Those persons who took the vaccine will not have a strong pleasurable response to opioids. Given that substance abuse is not contagious like measles, it is unlikely that many people would take an opioid vaccine, even if it was effective. Possibly in the future when you know your genome and whether you are prone to addiction, a vaccine will be valuable.

We have finally unlocked the genome for humans. Everyone has their own genetic makeup. One study claims that naltrexone works best for someone with a family history of alcoholism. Another study, indicates that a gene called HK2, "involved in dopaminergic activity in the brain, is more frequently found in drug addicts" (PNAS October 9, 2018 115 (41)). When I worked with schizophrenics, treating them with medications was a process of trial and error. More than 50 medications have been tested for cocaine abuse.

Sometime in the future we will unravel the genes related to being predisposed to addiction. If parents were told that their third child is prone to addiction, I expect that would lead to differences in how they were brought up.

Scientists have a procedure called CRISPR that allows for gene alteration. In the distant future we can expect various genetic-based illnesses to be eradicated. CRISPR is presently working on cures for sickle cell disease and blindness. Possibly, the predisposition to addiction can be altered.

Like many others, I noticed that alcoholics in treatment are heavy on smoking and coffee drinking. Consequently, I was surprised to discover that the chromosomes related to heavy drinking were very different from the ones related to heavy smoking (Deborah Hasin et al, "Genetics of Substance Use Disorders" in *Rethinking Substance Abuse*). Stopping caffeine can produce withdrawal symptoms such as fatigue and headaches. Too much caffeine can lead to insomnia, anxiety, and even cardiac arrhythmias (*Tufts Health & Nutrition Letter*, April, 2019). Fortunately, most people can control their use of caffeine.

At the present time, our knowledge of the pathways for addiction have not led to any breakthrough therapies. Medication-Assisted treatment was available in the 1970's with methadone. Naltrexone was available in the 1980's. Perhaps something new is just around the corner.

Although I intended to say very little about drugs and brain chemistry, I feel I need to say the following to correct what I believe are misconceptions. All of the following are related to the potential for both drug abuse and treatment:

1. Individual genes.
2. The combination of genes.
3. How the environment alters the expression of these genes including in the womb (epigenetics).
4. How the environment interacts with genes that are fully or partially expressed (penetrance).
5. How the body processes a substance (pharmacokinetics).
6. Some chemical processes increase reactions (i.e., more dopamine) while other chemical processes decrease reactions (i.e., less GABA).
7. The effect of nutrients on gene expression (nutrigenomics).
8. The role of phenocopies (traits that mimic a genetic quality).

"All genetic influence, we've learned, is context dependent and incredibly complex" (*Never Enough*, p. 187). Not only am I not an expert in addictions, I am far from an expert in genetics and physiology. Consequently, it is my <u>opinion</u>

that the explanations regarding brain chemistry and substance abuse as given in several of the books I have read are overly simplistic. I believe that future computer models will greatly improve our understanding of the chemical/physical processes involved with the taking of drugs (legal and illegal) and how they relate to individual differences.

Psychedelics

Psychedelics include LSD, MDMA (ecstasy), psilocybin (peyote), ayahuasca, ibogaine and ketamine. Strick regulation of these substances has delayed research as to their value to help people. Times are changing.

The *"Acid Test"* by Tom Shroder (2014) particularly deals with ecstasy and LSD as ways to treat post-traumatic stress syndrome. He talks about twenty-one subjects taking a single dose of ecstasy where everyone had a positive experience. In another experiment, 10 of 12 subjects who took ecstasy no longer merited a diagnosis of post-traumatic stress syndrome (PTSD) compared with 2 of 8 control subjects.

A Washington Post article written in 2017 (140, No. 265) sees ecstasy as a possible breakthrough for PTSD. Up to 20% of the soldiers returning from Iraq or Afghanistan suffer from PTSD. Using ecstasy on 107 patients, 67% a year later longer had PTSD.

Newsweek (August 23, 2018) reports psilocybin as a possibility for treatment-resistant depression. A 2016 study by New York University and Johns Hopkins reported that a single dose of psilocybin reduced symptoms of anxiety in cancer patients for eight months. The article says "Growing evidence suggests psychedelic substances, such as psilocybin, LSD, MDMA, ayahuasca, peyote and ibogaine, could be used to treat mental illnesses such as depression, anxiety and post-traumatic stress disorder in a controlled medical setting."

Ketamine is an anesthetic but is also a hallucinogen. Ketamine is being tried for depression, obsessive-compulsive disorder (OCD), Post Traumatic Stress Disorder (PTSD), and extreme anxiety (*Washington Post*, Feb 2, 2016). If it works for OCD there is a possibility that it will work for drug abuse.

Clearly, the addictions will be next for treatment with psychedelics. LSD had already been tried for alcoholism in the 1960's. In 2009, Johns Hopkins ran a pilot study treating 15 smoking volunteers with Cognitive Behavioral Therapy followed by 3 doses of psilocybin. Six months later, 12 persons were abstinent and one year later 10 were still abstinent. (No control group was used.)

While a graduate student at the University of Texas, I worked at a center for talking down people who were having a bad experience from LSD. I was usually able to quickly calm a person down as LSD increases a person's suggestibility. I expect that is true for other psychedelics. Consequently, it is import to determine if the psychological improvements under psychedelics are primarily the results of increased suggestibility. I remember when hypnosis was the primary therapy to quit smoking. Now I hardly ever hear of that therapy mentioned.

It has already been shown that persons taking LSD under favorable conditions rarely have bad "trips". There is even a study in the 1960's where seminary students took LSD. None of these students had a bad experience. Even Steve Jobs of Apple praised LSD. However, flashbacks can be a problem. Also, individual differences in responses to hallucinogens are common.

Peyote, ayahuasca and ibogaine are psychedelics that have been used within a religious or social setting. Again, group expectations with a psychedelic seem to promote good experiences and social bonding. I have never met an alcoholic who said it all started with communion!

Cannabidiol (CBD) comes from marijuana and is used for epilepsy. This is not the addictive substance (THC) in marijuana and we might discover a use for it in the treatment of addiction. According to *Consumer Reports*, May 2019, 63% report CBD to be "extremely or very effective" for reducing stress and anxiety. Also, 52% report CBD to be "extremely or very effective" for better sleep.

Nutritional Supplements

There are more books on nutrition than you can count. There are so many diet plans and theories that I subscribe to Tufts University *Health & Nutrition Letter*.

The Addiction Spectrum, 2018, by Paul Thomas and Jennifer Margulis advocates a holistic approach to recovery. They refer to a 2013 college research paper that "found that Oreo cookies were as addictive to rats as cocaine and morphine" (p. 65). This is a study that definitely needs replication. We know that chronic inflammation is related to many illnesses. Might it be related to substance abuse?

Recent research shows that our gut and brain are closely related. The neurotransmitter serotonin is found mostly in our digestive system. Sunlight and meditation increase your levels of serotonin (Young, *Journal of Psychiatric Neuroscience*, 2007, 32(6)). Eating foods rich in tyrosine (almonds, bananas, fish, etc.) and reducing your sugar intake increases dopamine. According to Bob Roehr, drinking alcohol causes a gut microbe imbalance that may lead to liver disease (The Microbiome: Your Inner Eco System, *Scientific American* E-book, 2019).

Folate is related to the production of neurotransmitters. "A deficiency of folate can not only lead to depression but also hinder recovery from it" (Hara Estoff Marano, *Psychology Today*, Feb. 2019, p.34). Furthermore, "about a third of people with major depression have evidence of inflammation somewhere in the body" (Edward Bullmore, *Psychology Today*, Feb. 2019, p.53). Not surprisingly, steroids that reduce inflammation often improve a person's mood.

A few addiction treatment centers are using Nicotinamide Adenine Dinucleotide (NAD) with intravenous hookups (about ten days) to treat addiction.

NAD is involved with cell mitochondria and metabolism. Studies have shown it to make mice appear younger and is useful for jet lag in humans. Those administering this procedure say it works best on alcohol and opiate users. Unfortunately, I could not find any studies that use a sham control group with an IV hook-up to compare this with its actual treatment. Some users of this technique say it makes detoxification easy and reduces cravings. Clearly, we need more research on this therapy.

High Tech Therapies

High Tech therapies include transcranial magnetic stimulation (TMS) used mostly for severe depression. One study found repetitive TMS to reduce nicotine cravings and another study to reduce cocaine use (Gorelick et al, *Annals of New York Academy of Science*, 2014, 1327). The University of Louisville has used this therapy on over 200 high-functioning autistic children and reported that about 90% of them showed improvement (*Washington Post*, Jan 13, 2015). Neuroscientists at the University of Texas found TMS to facilitate cognitive therapy. A devise available to the general public, called Thync uses transcranial pulsed ultrasound to produce relaxation/calmness.

Magnetic resonance therapy, a variation of transcranial magnetic stimulation, is still experimental and has been used for autism and post-traumatic stress syndrome.

High frequency stimulation of the subthalamic nucleus demonstrated reduced heroin use in rats and will hopefully produce similar results in humans (Internet - practicalpainmanagement.com/treatments/addiction-medicine ...).

Functional Magnetic Resonance Imaging (fMRI) done in real time exposes a person to their own brain activity. This neurofeedback technique would allow a person to modify brain activity directly. Feedback from the anterior cingulate cortex (ACC) has been used to modify pain and depression (*Scientific American Mind,* 2013, Mar./Apr.). A variation of this neurofeedback technique has promise for addiction.

The FDA approved a new device that eases opioid withdrawal by sending signals to the cranial and occipital nerves through skin behind the ear (*FDA News Release,* Nov. 15, 2017, Internet).

Virtual Reality has been effective in working with phobias. For example, people afraid of flying can learn to relax in an airplane by first doing it with virtual reality. The technique used is called desensitization. Persons face their fears little by little. At the same time pleasant stimuli such as soothing music can facilitate this process.

Virtual reality can also be used to simulate situations likely to trigger drug cravings. The technique of exposure and response prevention can be used with virtual reality to eventually extinguish these cravings. Incompatible behaviors can also be taught to prevent relapses.

Researchers at Stanford University discovered that "Using just activity in the nucleus accumbens, the team could correctly identify 77 percent of the patients who relapsed by three months" (Futurity.org, Jan. 2, 2019). Assuming a 50% relapse rate, they exceeded chance by 27%. This study was based on male veterans and definitely needs to be replicated by a disinterested party. Another study done at the University of California, San Diego "found that brain imaging performed at the end of treatment for methamphetamine abuse predicted which patients would relapse during the following 12 months" (*Scientific American*, Mar. 2018).

Home Treatment

We presently have inpatient and outpatient care. People can be treated in their own homes for addiction or other types of mental illness or dysfunctional behaviors. Physical and occupational therapy are often done entirely at the client's home. I see no reason why some counselors would not want to save on office rental by seeing people in their homes. "Aware Recovery Care" in Connecticut has an in-home rehabilitation program for $38,000 per year. They say 64% complete the program with 72% staying abstinent. (Note: .64 X .72 = 46%)

One of the problems with inpatient treatment is whether the client's new behaviors will transfer to back home. It is relatively easy to stay clean when you are surrounded by staff in an environment where no drugs are available. AA and NA give group support in the community. So does living in a drug free environment such as sober house.

The Internet isn't exactly high tech but is now available for providing treatment. This is especially promising for small towns and rural areas. The Internet provides for one-to-one counseling as well as goal setting and relapse prevention techniques. Some preliminary studies have found it to help people reduce their drinking (*Drug and Alcohol Review*, 2009, 28(1)). Telepsychiatry can provide services to people in outlying areas. This can involve video sessions or texting. The Recovery Line is an automated, computer-based intervention based on cognitive behavioral therapy designed for patients in methadone maintenance. Based on 22 studies, computerized therapy for anxiety and depression appears to be effective (PLoS One, 2010, 5(10)). A virtual (computer program) therapist called ELIZA was created in the 1960's. Surprisingly, so little has happened since.

Replacing Drug Highs with Natural Highs

I have my own idea of what I think is underutilized approach to addiction. My father was an alcoholic but had neither a stressful life or hung out with heavy drinkers. He did, however, like to drive exceedingly fast. Many drug addicts are young males. Risk taking is known to increase one's chances of becoming an addict. So here is my hypothesis (admittedly not new) – replace a drug high with an adrenaline high. How about sky diving? George H.W. Bush went sky diving on his 90th birthday! Sky diving would give a whole new meaning to "getting high". White water rafting is another exciting sport. I have been a snow skier for over 50 years. I find it exhilarating. In college, my specialty in gymnastics was the high bar. People would ask me if I found this event to be scary. My response was that it is scary the way a roller coaster is scary. It is a fun scary.

The relapse of an addict is often considered to be related to a trigger/classical conditioning. A manic-depressive relative of mine will sometimes stop taking her medication. Is there is a trigger to stop taking medication? Apparently, she stops her medication because she misses the feeling of being on a manic high.

I am far from the first person to associate drug use with risk taking and sensation seeking. Anna Rose Childress recommends that "early prevention might encourage the pursuit of highly stimulating nondrug activities that are prosocial – for example, volunteering with paramedics or firefighters, or in a hospital emergency room" (*Rethinking Substance Abuse, p. 54*). The Substance Use Risk Profile Scale given to teenagers considers impulsive and sensation seeking behaviors to indicate potential drug users. Replacing a drug high with an adrenaline high might require virtual reality where someone can safely do bungy jumping without leaving the facility.

Unfortunately, many addicts have too much adrenaline. They are often people who have been traumatized (PTSD). Consequently, only a small group of addicts would benefit by the rush of adrenalin. What is most important is that people with too much adrenalin and people who do not get enough adrenalin should not be in the same room together, let alone in the same treatment program. Individualized treatment is one thing, but I cannot expect a treatment center to take someone skydiving or white-water rafting while their comrades are going to meditation and yoga to calm down.

I believe that many addicts could benefit from the feel of powerful positive emotions. Seeking a natural emotional high as a replacement for a drug high is not a new idea. However, it has usually been treated as an adjunct to addiction treatment, not its primary focus. Charismatic religion and even AA and NA can produce strong positive emotions. Religious involvement contributes to long-term abstinence. People in the Gospel Tent at Jazz Fest get very emotional. Young people seem especially prone to emotion at concerts. Music and the arts are designed to produce emotion. Singing and dancing release endorphins and raise the threshold for pain (*Evolutionary Psychology*, 2012, 10(4)). Exercise such as running is also known to release endorphins. Endorphins trigger a positive feeling in the body, similar to that of morphine. Cognitive therapy is great for people with distorted thinking but I believe many addicts need a more emotional/physical solution.

Evolutionary Psychology

According to the Harvard Medical School (*Overcoming Addiction*, 2017), about 13% of heroin users become addicted. This figure is probably reliable as it also applies to rats. Why would there be such a high rate of genes/chromosomes that make someone prone to addiction? Suppose a few thousand years ago you are with a group of 17 persons hunting for food. You come across some mushrooms. The group leader says "Who will eat a mushroom to see if it is poisonous?" Any normal person thinks "I could get killed." Every group needs a person who says "That looks exciting!" If 13% of the people have the genetics that make them fearless and/or enjoy excitement, a group of 17 has better than a 90% chance that they have such a person. Remember, some addicts have reward insufficiency. The ordinary things that make most people happy are not enough for them. I could be wrong about an addictive gene that makes someone fearless and/or a sensation seeker. However, answering this evolutionary mystery is sure to create insight on how to treat people genetically prone to addiction.

Some people believe that a certain percentage of people are destined to be overweight because they will survive a famine. On the other hand, it is unlikely that one-third of the population has this predisposition. Consequently, we can expect a small percentage of obese persons to be resistant to most forms of weight loss. The same might hold true for a small percentage of addicts. Some day we will know who these people are by their genomes and personal history.

Many people are skeptical about tampering with someone's genetics. It is difficult to predict the consequences. It is possible that addicts have a lot in common with people with "the right stuff". Perhaps, Neil Armstrong and John Glenn chose the excitement and danger of space travel over drugs. We will always need soldiers and fire fighters.

Caveats Regarding New Research

Given the low success rates of current treatment practices, I believe it is better to put more money into research and less into treatment. I also believe there is promise in the use of psychedelics to treat the addictions because of the emotions they produce and the possibility of seeing the world differently. I expect you will hear a lot about this in the next ten years. However, you need to keep in mind the following caveats regarding new research.

(1) The Hawthorne Effect – Someone might go to a factory and say that if they had more light, they could do a better job. So, they improve the lighting and sure enough, production goes up. At a similar factory they are told that less light would make them more relaxed and thereby improve production. So, they reduce the lighting and sure enough, production goes up. The Hawthorn Effect is a type of placebo effect. People get what they expect.

(2) Researcher bias – Who would not like being the originator of the latest and greatest discovery? Pharmaceutical companies do most of their own research or use a trusted researcher as in trusted to want more money for their next project.

(3) Research journals favor positive results. A study that shows no difference between two treatments is less likely to get published than one that does.

(4) Regression to the mean - Chance and variable factors influence every study. A large effect is likely to be smaller on replication. I have a stock market model that shows you can make money by selling after a large single day jump in the stock market and by buying after a large single day drop.

(5) No one likes replicating someone else's work to see if the results are consistent. NIDA should fund this. Psychologists tried to replicate 100 studies. Only 36% were in line with the original findings (*Scientific American*, Oct. 2018)

(6) Statistical Errors – Using R-package "statcheck" on eight major psychology journals from 1985 to 2013, researchers found half of the papers with at least one probability value in error. One in eight papers contained a value that may have altered the conclusions (Nuijten et al, *Behavior Research Methods*, 2016, 48(4)). In 2014, the *Lancet* reported that an estimated 85 percent of investments in biomedical research is wasted (*Scientific American*, Oct. 2018)

(7) If the new treatment involves the brain, unless you or the person explaining it to you has a Ph.D. in neurology, ignore any and all neurological explanations.

The bottom line is do not get too excited about the hype that goes with new research. Much of it is likely to wear off in time. Remember that psychedelics increase suggestibility. A control group needs to be given the same psychedelic as the experimental group but with different instructions such as "We are assessing how many people have bad trips" as opposed to "We think this is a cure for addictions."

As you probably noticed, I am a believer in meta-analysis. This is when a group of researchers look over several similar studies to form conclusions. Hopefully, these researchers were not involved in the original studies. These studies first look for methodological or statistical errors. While at Brainerd State Hospital, we encountered several studies that showed nicotinic acid to be helpful in the treatment of schizophrenia. We tried this approach to no avail. Later, we discovered that the studies we encountered were done by persons who were all part of the same group. We were duped by thinking multiple studies could not be wrong.

Research versus Program Evaluation

Consider the following hypothetical example. A company is looking to hire people for a job that involves heavy labor. They are thinking of hiring young people; however, they are unsure that this is the best way to go. They decide to look at the research that has been done.

The first study they encounter involves a large random sample. The study concludes that there is only a small positive correlation between strength and age. (Note: correlations vary from -1 to +1. Zero implies no relationship and -1 and +1 are perfect negative and positive correlations.)

The second study looks only at men and finds a moderate correlation between strength and age.

The third study looks only at males between the ages of 5 and 20 and finds a strong correlation between strength and age.

The fourth study looks at persons over the age of 60 and finds a negative correlation between strength and age.

All of the above studies are valid. Unfortunately, none of the studies limit themselves to people between the ages of 18 and 65; the target age this company intends to interview. Of course, they could interview everyone and give them a strength test and use that as their criterion. However, this choice carries a heavy price tag compared with first preselecting job applicants. Perhaps they might discover, too late, that what they really want is stamina, not absolute strength. Looking at stamina, women do not necessarily fall behind the men. Plus, there are potential legal ramifications if they discriminate against women and/or the elderly.

The experimental designs of most research projects are limited to answering specific questions regarding the strength of relationships. Program evaluation helps administrators make decisions in the real world. I have seen numerous research studies that show method 'A' is statistically significant to method 'B'. I have never seen a research study that concluded in the abstract that "Although method 'A' is better than method 'B', ($p<.01$), method 'B' is more cost efficient."

NIDA, SAMHSA and others have produced estimates on how much alcohol and other addictions are costing the United States on a yearly basis. I have never seen any valid estimates on how much drug prevention and drug treatment are saving us on a yearly basis. NIDA says "According to several conservative estimates, every dollar invested in addiction treatment programs yields a return of between $4 and $7 in reduced drug-related crime, criminal justice costs, and theft. When savings related to healthcare are included, total savings can exceed costs by a ratio of 12 to 1. Major savings to the individual and to society also stem from fewer interpersonal conflicts; greater workplace productivity; and fewer drug-related accidents, including overdoses and deaths" (Internet – "Is drug addiction treatment worth its cost"). Giving first responders naloxone is cost effective. Addiction treatment instead of jail is cost effective. The savings of addiction treatment by itself is unknown.

Not only is the savings of addiction treatment unknown, it will always be unknown. The economists that says addiction treatment is a cost savings are probably the same ones that say going to college will increase your income. There is absolutely no evidence that going to college will increase your income. To do so would involve taking a sample of high school graduates and randomly assigning some to college and some who must not go to college. (I actually suggested this to the Bill Gates Foundation.) By the same token, to measure the savings of addiction treatment we would have to randomly assign some substance abusers to either treatment or to no treatment and follow them for several years. This is never going to happen. The best we can do is compare different treatments.

This is another reason for putting MBA's in charge of state addiction programs. MBA's have an understanding of sunk costs, overhead, inflation, amortizing, discounting, and various other economic concepts. MBA's understand they would need to make hard decisions that may involve reducing funds to programs that help people.

I believe the gains we have made in treating cancer and heart disease over the last 40 years have paid back most of our investments in research. Can we say the same about substance abuse? On the other hand, we have not made any significant gains in the treatment of Alzheimer's. However, as baby boomers get older, we can expect those costs to go up. Do we expect substance abuse costs to continue upwards? I am not sure about substance abuse but I expect addictions to electronic devices to sharply increase. Where is the money for that?

I have done program evaluation for a psychiatric hospital, for a correctional program and for several educational programs. People running programs cannot wait for the research to be in. They must make daily decisions on the most relevant information at hand. All of these decisions involve money. Administrators are also in the best position to know what additional data would be the most helpful. I know that when I worked for a psychiatric hospital, I would have loved a paper and pencil test that told me which schizophrenics would get better with tranquilizers. Instead, all we had was trial and error.

The federal government is giving millions of dollars for research on opioid addiction but nothing for program evaluation. I believe the principal reason is ignorance. Even the man on the street knows what research is. You try a drug or a procedure on a group of people and measure the results. Most people probably even know that research uses a control group or placebo. Studies that show positive results become "evidence-based".

Almost no one understands program evaluation. First of all, the medical model rarely uses it. For one thing, sick people usually know when they are well. Plus, many people get over illnesses without any medical assistance. Our bodies often heal themselves.

Counselors have no interest in program evaluation. Not only does program evaluation mean extra work but it has the potential of making them look bad. Furthermore, program evaluation opens the door for people without advanced degrees to demonstrate that they can counsel as well as those with advanced degrees.

As I said earlier, there are several reasons for the state to do referral and follow-up. Scale 1 of the MMPI measures hypochondriasis and scale 3 measures hysteria. People who score high on these scales usually have strong physical concerns or ailments. These are people who somaticize. They include hypochondriacs and people who are psychologically clueless. How do these people respond to addiction treatment? You will probably never have a research study on these people because they make up such a small proportion of substance abusers. With state referral offices giving everyone the MMPI and doing follow-up, it is only a matter of time before we have enough of these people to see how they fare under standard treatment. The efforts of the states doing referral and follow-up fall under program evaluation. Researchers with high skill levels and highly controlled settings can gain valuable information, but we have to deal with what we know now. NIDA should fund research but the states should spend their money on developing a system of feedback (program evaluation).

My Experience with Treatment Centers

Treatment centers make various claims. Seven of my sample of 26 treatment centers use testimonials. Have you ever read a bad testimonial? I would like to pay someone to submit a bad testimonial just to see if it ends up on their website. On the other hand, I would bet the people who give testimonials have a lower relapse rate than most. These people have put a lot on the line with their name, picture and glowing reviews.

Whenever I go to a health fair, I ask someone from an addiction treatment center for the success rate of their center. Sometimes I get a blank stare but usually they pull a figure out of the air, such as 80% for those who stick with the program. True story: I gave a talk at a VA hospital once. I said I had a one hundred percent success rate for those who stick with my program. They thought I was joking. I said "No, I am serious." So, what was my program? I sat across a desk from my client, looked the person in the eye and said "don't drink." Everybody that followed my program got better. Fortunately, we have something called Motivational Interviewing to help people stick with the program. That is part of the treatment process.

Sometimes I ask someone from a treatment center "What percent of your clients were you unable to locate?" This always gets a blank stare as apparently no one else has ever asked this question. People move out of state. People die. People go to jail. People end up in other treatment centers. Anyone doing serious follow-up should be able to tell you the percent of clients they were unable to locate. It would be helpful if someone made an effort to find as many as possible of those persons who were not included in a report giving relapse rates to see how much they differ from the others. The Assisi Bridge House in Louisiana has a simple one-page report that includes all of the vital follow-up statistics you would expect from a treatment facility (Appendix 2).

Follow-Up Evaluations

The collection of relapse rates requires home visits. My own research made that clear years ago! At Brainerd State Hospital, for every admission, we sent a significant other such as a spouse, relative or friend, the Patient Adjustment and Role Skills (PARS) form to rate the person's condition on entering treatment. The PARS measured Interpersonal Involvement, Agitation-Depression, Confusion, Anxiety, Alcohol or Drug Use, Socially Active, Household Management, Employment, and Parenthood Skills. Three months and six months after treatment, we re-sent the PARS to measure improvement. We initially got an 82% response upon hospital admission. At six months after discharge the response rate dropped to 42%.

Eighty-eight percent (88%) of our chemically dependent discharges were reported to be improved with 62% rated abstinent by a significant other. Clearly, significant others are more biased than expected. Of course, we did not know the abstinent rate for non-responders. When I was chairman of the Research Committee of Psychologists in Public Service, we did a special study where pairs of psychologists rated incoming psychiatric patients and later visited them at their homes in the community for a second rating. We found improvements to be minimal with over half of the former patients looking the same. According to significant others, 93% of our former psychiatric patients showed improvement. Who am I to believe? Should I believe pairs of trained psychologists or significant others? Face to face visits give us the additional information of appearance and body language. We can often get consensual validation from someone else in the home. We can ask additional questions if it appears that the subject is not being honest.

According to the Hazelden website, "70.18% reported abstinence at nine months follow-up survey between July 2016 and June 2917". Response rates were about 70%. **Trying to follow-up all addiction treatment clients does not work!** The correct procedure is to select a random sample and hunt them down until you can do **face to face** interviews with over 90% of your sample. Hazelden only needs to do this study once to see if I am right. If I am right, the study I am suggesting will significantly lower their rates of abstinence.

I created many surveys when I spent three years evaluating educational programs in Texas. It is difficult to create surveys that will produce valid responses. One study found that people who exercised were less likely (26%) to become depressed "but only when the exercise was measured objectively using a tracking device, not when people self-reported how much exercise they performed" *JAMA Psychiatry*, Jan. 23 online).

I recommend the following study. Create a free workshop to help people lose weight. Teach them about healthy diets (no sodas, less red meat, etc.), environmental changes (no food in sight, smaller plates, etc.) and the consequences of losing weight (look better, live longer, etc.). Weigh everyone and then send them home. Three months later, mail or email them a survey asking them the following question – How closely have you been following your program to lose weight? Answers include (1) Faithfully, (2) Most of the time, (3) Often, (4) Sometimes, and (5) Rarely. What they do not know is that within the next few days you are going to show up at their homes with a scale! Now we can correlate their survey responses with actual results. What do you think will be the correlation between the survey and actual weight loss? Will the actual weight loss look less promising than the survey results? In addition, we will also show up at the homes of those people who did not respond to the survey. How do you think they will differ?

Face to face visits allow for consensual validation, that is, getting someone else to verify what the former client/patient says. Before visiting the person, you should let him know that you would prefer a significant other at the follow-up interview, preferably the same person who was with him during the diagnosis and referral process.

In-home follow-up also gives the interviewer a chance to see if persons living with the former client are helpful in keeping the client clean. If people close to the person are drug users themselves, his chance of success are slim. Although if is difficult to make any snap judgment on how supportive are those who surround a former client, any clues are better than the none received from a telephone or Internet follow-up. Even with a person who lives alone, the condition of his home can be telling (e.g., dishes piled up in the sink, food not put away).

I recommend that follow-up on addiction treatment be done twice - once at six months after treatment and again at one year after treatment. Appendix 3 presents a sample of the kind of questions that could be asked during a follow-up interview. Follow-up is costly but small in comparison to the cost of treatment. Furthermore, follow-up is based on a stratified sample, not on everybody. Stratified means that you want to include the right proportion of certain variables such as inpatient versus outpatient therapy, first admissions versus readmissions, and also include socioeconomic status. Furthermore, you probably should limit yourself to a select number of treatment centers and choose different treatment centers each year.

With standardized follow-up, we will be able to spend more time looking at improvement instead of focusing on abstinence. However, if I am correct, we will find a strong correlation between abstinence and other improvements. In other words, I expect that programs that produce the most abstinence will also produce the most improvement in their clients including those not abstinent.

The primary reason there are measures of improvement I do not trust is because these measures often lack reliability or validity. For example, having a job might rely more on the person helping a client than on the client. Furthermore, measures of improvement might fluctuate over time even more than the measure of abstinence. In any case, one follow-up is insufficient. It is also possible that being part of a special research project biases the results. People who know they are part of a study might do better. This problem will no longer exist when the state takes random samples for follow-up.

If the state is going to do referrals and follow-up, they will need to collect some statistics on the treatment centers such as:

1. Staff – total numbers broken down by degrees & certifications
2. Staff turnover rates (known to be high for addiction treatment)
3. Cost per day and length of stay
4. Typical number of clients by inpatient/outpatient
5. Services offered
6. Funding – insurance, Medicaid, etc.

At Brainerd State Hospital we keep various statistics for the mentally ill and chemically dependent including the following: (See Appendix 4 for more)

	Mentally ill	Chemically Dependent
1. Readmission within 6 months after discharge	22%	32%
2. Reported to be better 6 months after hospitalization by a significant other in the community	93%	88%
3. Ex-patients reporting to be Improved 1 month after hospitalization.	85%	85%

We also had patients fill out a form upon discharge telling us which services helped them the most using rank ordering. Every program, including recreation, received a number one ranking by at least one person. Without feedback how would we know that patients who left against medical advice did as well as the others or that women prefer medications over men. Our efforts at evaluation helped Brainerd State Hospital became one of only seven multi-service hospitals nationwide to become accredited.

I don't blame treatment centers for not collecting relapse rates. Minnesota created a statute in the '90's that required addiction treatment centers to collect data upon admission and again six months later. It failed. Small treatment centers did not have the resources and large centers discovered that hunting down people was harder than expected. As of 2001, less than two-thirds of the treatment centers submitted even baseline data. That is one reason why I believe it is the responsibility of the states to collect data on relapses using sampling. Plus, they are less biased. These same referral centers can use that data for recommending a treatment center after a diagnostic assessment. Furthermore, the states have the money to do assessments and follow-up as long as they limit the money on evidence-based treatment.

This doesn't mean that treatment facilities should not also do their own follow-up. A treatment facility is not only interested in what works for them but in helping former clients. Hazelden has a program called MORE (My Ongoing Recovery Experience) that provides 18 months of support after treatment.

As a minimum, treatment centers can use an app. Sparkite founder Lauren Stahl says "App users receive a weekly quality-of-life survey to help treatment facilities really understand what is happening with clients once they are discharged from treatment. We provide the facilities with the data from these surveys so they can measure addiction recovery on a client as well as facility level."

If one's treatment included one-on-one counseling, clients should be able to rate their counselor. There is data that clients who rate their counselors higher do better. This could be done on the Internet with computers doing all of the work including putting the responses into a database where reports can be generated automatically (See Appendix 5 for an example). Once several clients have rated the same counselor, a counselor profile can be generated. Program evaluation can help us determine the types of counseling that work best and for whom. It can also indicate counselors who are not cutting it.

As previously mentioned, the NIDA believes drug addiction is a chronic illness like diabetes, hypertension, and asthma. Most people with one of these diseases are referred to a specialist from their primary physician. Therefore, their primary physician can assist with follow-up and verify the work of the specialist. Less than 3% of referrals to addiction treatment centers comes from primary physicians. Consequently, we cannot rely on a person's primary physician to either provide follow-up or to verify the success of those persons who were in addiction treatment.

The states should eventually do an assessment of living facilities (sober houses) for persons who were addicted and are now trying to keep clean/sober with the help of their peers. Unfortunately, just as there are treatment centers that exist primarily as money makers, the same is true for living centers for former substance abusers. As previously mentioned, there are many self-help groups for addicts. In the best of all worlds they should be evaluated like paid treatment programs but are clearly low on the priority list.

Prevention

Whereas the gains from addiction treatment are small, the gains from drug prevention programs are unknown. SAMHSA has a list of evidenced-based prevention programs. So why do I disagree? Because, based on my limited research, drug prevention programs never have a suitable control group. It seems reasonable to people not familiar with research that if a school did not previously have a drug prevention program, they can compare students who took such a program with students who received nothing or perhaps some sort of lecture. A suitable control group requires just as much time and effort as the real program. The control group should also be given the expectation of being effective.

Here is what I recommend for a drug prevention control group. Students be given a CD on "rewiring the brain" or something similar. These students should be told that it has been proven that people who complete this CD are resistant to becoming addicted to drugs. CDs on how drugs affect the brain are full of neurological explanations. Students (and many adults) will not know that even if the neurology is correct, that doesn't make the treatment effective. The best thing about this control group is that a CD on the brain will cost less than twenty dollars whereas most drug prevention programs cost well over $100 per student.

Determining trends in drug use requires several observations. According to Statistical Process Control, you can be confident that change is occurring if seven or more consecutive observations in time are heading up or down, or if seven or more consecutive observations are above or below average. The use of e-cigarettes (vaping) has steadily increased among high school students from 1.5% in 2011 to 20.8% in 2018 (U.S. Center for Disease Control and Prevention). This is a reliable increase. However, New Orleans law enforcement takes credit every year crime goes down and blame factors beyond their control, such as the infiltration of drugs, for years when crime goes up. Remember, getting three heads in a row is not sufficient evidence that the coin is biased.

Identifying areas of high drug use can be done with police and hospital records. The University of California Institute for Prediction Technology forecasts opioid overdose based on Google searches (*Scientific American*, January, 2019). They claim their model explains 72% of the overdose statistics.

What are some of the factors that make a person more likely to become an addict? John Petraitis et al surveys the literature on adolescent substance use

(*Psychological Bulletin*, 1995, Vol. 17) and comes up with the following factors:

1. Social/Interpersonal – Peer influence, lack of parental controls, etc.
2. Cultural/Attitudinal – Inadequate schools, high crime, poverty, etc.
3. Intrapersonal – Impulsive, low self-esteem, ADHD, etc.

I am going to save you a whole chapter of studies that answers what factors go with drug abuse. Why? Because <u>everything bad that can happen to a person increases the chance of drug addiction</u>. This list includes physical, sexual and emotional abuse, being a crime victim, early trauma and Post Traumatic Stress Disorder, physical pain, poverty and divorce, learning disorders, ADHD, anxiety, depression and other mental illnesses. Some people see drug use as their only hope for feeling good.

One problem with looking for antecedents for drug abuse is that these are often the same factors that will increase a person's chances for ending up in corrections or needing the help of a counselor. We have always known that reducing poverty diminishes a number of ailments. Programs for early childhood development and early intervention have always been helpful for preventing future problems. Programs that get children into healthy activities such as sports and the arts keep them out of trouble. Everyone needs good nutrition and exercise.

David Sheff (*Clean*, 2013) has a chapter on "Helping Kids Grow Up". Outside of practiced strategies for handling drug situations and a code word text for parents to call the child's cell phone to come home, over 90% of the activities he endorses are not specific to drug addiction. I am all for teaching life skills such as communication, anger management, conflict resolution and assertive training. I believe in building parent-child relationships. Everyone needs to develop healthy activities such as sports, the arts, or belonging to an interest group. However, when funding a drug prevention program, the first question you should ask is "Would this still be a good idea if we did not have a drug problem?" If the answer is "yes", then I have a problem with using money from your state office on substance abuse or from an organization like the National Institute of Drug Abuse. The system I am proposing of referral and follow-up would be unnecessary without a drug problem. Consequently, I believe my idea for a diagnosis and follow-up system for addiction should get first funding from agencies that deal with drug abuse.

Not surprisingly, the traits of people prone to addiction include impulsive, defiant, nonattentive and poor cognitive/reasoning skills. Those persons least likely to be a substance abuser are conscientious, attentive, and show foresight/planning abilities. Among young people, Openness (i.e., interested in trying new things) and

Extraversion (likely to be part of a group) are also somewhat more prone to become a substance abuser.

With so many factors increasing a person's chance of becoming an addict, what do we choose to be part of drug prevention program? Should we center prevention around educating children on the facts about drug abuse? Certainly, some information about drug abuse could be helpful. However, ask yourself if telling teenagers the following facts would be helpful:

(1) The chances of you becoming addicted after your first hit of heroin or cocaine is highly unlikely. You would probably need to take the drug several times.
(2) Some people take an opioid such as heroin on a regular basis and have never been in any sort of trouble.
(3) Many drug users have quit on their own. (Note: There are few studies on these people.)
(4) Psychedelic drugs such a peyote, ayahuasca and ibogaine have been a part of various cultures with few bad effects.
(5) Using alcohol in moderation is a modern invention. Anthropologists say that primitive cultures typically used alcohol to become intoxicated.
(6) A recent study of people over 50 showed that those who drank alcohol in moderation lived longer than those who did not drink at all.

Some drug education is helpful. In any case, nearly all of the addiction experts agree that education is one of the least effective methods in the treatment of addiction.

The following is an opinion of mine – Do not write a book on addiction that deals with both children and adults. Why? Because the overwhelming number of experts already agree that alcohol, cigarettes, marijuana and various street drugs are not good for children and teenagers. The same could be said for expectant mothers. We already know that the sooner you get involved with drugs, the more problems you are likely to have. I would bet that 'A' and 'B' students in high school also use their cell phones, the Internet, and television less than the lower grade students. Even medicine has specialists for babies and children. I have read that couples that have more sex get along better. Do you think this will work for teenagers?

Not only are recreational drugs bad for children and teenagers, we are not sure about the effects of various medications on young people. It all starts at childbirth. Fentanyl is an epidural. What are the effects on the new baby? Is Adderall the best choice for ADHD in children? Do anxious and depressed children need the same medications given to adults?

I have another opinion – just about anything pleasurable can become an addiction. You can be addicted to golf, watching sports, gossiping, exercising, going to garage sales, etc. Consequently, one of the best ways to keep from becoming an addict is to avoid fun! The Addiction Spectrum refers to how addicted someone is. You can also have a spectrum on addictions that vary from serious to benign. Heroin, Meth and gambling are serious addictions. Fishing, exercise and crossword puzzles are benign addictions.

How do you know if you have a benign addiction? My wife and I exercise regularly three times a week. If we can come up with a good excuse to not exercise, we are elated. If we were addicted to exercise, we would feel uncomfortable missing a day. More than likely we would try to make up what we missed.

Propaganda

Whereas many drug prevention programs mention education, I have not found a single one that mentions propaganda. According to the dictionary, "propaganda is information, especially of a biased or misleading nature, used to promote or publicize a particular political cause or point of view." My own definition of propaganda is "promoting an idea by appealing to emotions that are not directly related to the idea." For example, what does a horse and a dog have to do with beer? Of course, I am referring to a Super Bowl favorite ad. When I ran my "Quit Smoking" group, I brought in various cigarette ads. My favorite was "For the taste of Springtime, smoke Salems." Does filling your lungs with smoke remind you of Springtime? Some people think that Joe Camel was created to appeal to young people.

Hitler was a big believer in propaganda. He has said that one should minimize appealing to the rational mind. He also said "By the skillful and sustained use of propaganda, one can make a people see even heaven as hell or an extremely wretched life as paradise." Hitler was able to lead an advanced nation into war.

If you believe in "evidenced based" methods, nothing compares with propaganda. Why? I can say this in one word – advertising. Advertising is often piloted in limited areas. Ads that work go nationwide. Those that don't are dropped. Advertising is evidenced based because the evidence is in dollars. No one cares how unrelated an ad is to the product if it brings in money. Will the right toothpaste really help you with the opposite sex? Pay attention to the next 20 ads you see. How often are you telling yourself "I didn't know that"? Very few ads are educational.

"Just say no" is not propaganda. Repetition is the only thing going for it; and yes, repetition does have power. If you want a song to be popular, it helps to have a "hook" that is often repeated. However, the ad that says "This is your brain and this is your brain on drugs" with the picture of an egg frying in a pan is definitely propaganda.

It taps into your emotions. The clever phrase "hijacks your brain" is also propaganda because the phrase is pejorative. It is used for heroin but not for buprenorphine. Perhaps we should say buprenorphine "restores" the brain.

The Twelve-Step program and others often use phrases to motivate their clients such as "One day at a time" and "Fake it 'till you make it". This is a close cousin of propaganda as these phrases often tap into your emotions. Do you remember the book, "Everything I Need to Know, I Learned in Kindergarten" by Robert Fulgham? Here are a few quotes from this book:

(A) "You may never have proof of your importance but you are more important than you think. There are always those who couldn't do without you. The rub is that you don't always know who."
(B) "It doesn't matter what you say you believe – it only matters what you do."
(C) "Sticks and stones may break our bones, but words will break our hearts."
(D) "It wasn't in books. It wasn't in church. What I needed to know was out there in the world."
(E) "If the dream is held close to the heart, and imagination is applied to what there is close at hand. Everything is still possible."

Aphorisms have power, especially with repetition, but I am a bigger believer in skill training which is often included in drug prevention and treatment programs. Decision making, assertive training and communication skills are helpful for everybody. I believe that learning social and psychological skills should be part of everyone's education, not just for drug prevention.

"Just say no" would be more effective if it was a part of assertive training. A major technique of assertive training is the "broken record". For example, if you are returning an item to a store for your money back and the clerk tries to talk you out of it, you reply to every objection with something like "I understand but I just want my money back". Assertive training involves not only role playing but trying out a real example and returning to the group to discuss how it went.

Active listening is a communications method that works for the general public as well as counselors. Paraphrasing what you heard is a major part of active listening. Paraphrasing lets the person speaking know that you are paying attention. Active listening also uses "I' messages to express your feelings and opinions.

Conflict resolution is a powerful skill that friends and family of substance abusers can learn. There are many sources on the steps of conflict resolution. The six steps I used in the 1970's were:

(1) Air out feelings –
  (A) Use active listening with "I" messages.
  (B) Avoid any judgments
(2) State desires and intentions –
  (A) State agreement to resolve the problem.
  (B) State general desires and intentions.
  (C) State specific desires and intentions.
  (D) Note mutual goals.
(3) Define the problem
  (A) Stick to the present situation, one problem at a time.
  (B) Talk about behaviors and events, not persons and personalities.

(C) Determine agreed upon facts and assumptions.

(D) What additional information would be helpful?

(4) Generate ideas –

(A) Don't make initial judgments.

(B) Expand on the idea and/or suggest alterations.

(C) Look for a mutually acceptable solution.

(D) Compromise.

(5) Determine a course of action –

(A) Obtain commitments of who is to do what by when.

(B) Show some latitude.

(6) Evaluate your plan.

(A) Use agreed upon measurable criteria.

(B) Have an alternative plan.

(C) Be willing to renegotiate if necessary.

Drugs in Moderation

When it comes to drug use, the following statistics are important:

(1) The number/percent of the population that use the drug.
(2) The percent that become addicted, that is, their drug use creates more problems than is solves.
(3) The number/percent of deaths the drug creates.
(4) The advantages of using the drug.
(5) The percent of people who use the drug in moderation.

We have known since the 1950's that there are people who use heroin without serious consequences. We know that people use alcohol, marijuana, and even nicotine (smoking) in moderation. I have never read a book on opioids that discusses using it in moderation. For one thing, a person who uses opioids in moderation is not likely to write a book. Plus, it would be difficult if not impossible to do a survey on opioid use in moderation given that the activity is illegal. On the other hand, we know that a sizable number of people have taken opioids for pain without abusing them. We also know that many opioid deaths are from taking fentanyl. I assume we can safely eliminate fentanyl as a drug to take in moderation.

Very few books seriously discuss the advantages of drugs. We know that alcohol promotes sociability and is good for the heart in moderation. Marijuana is good for cancer patients who become nauseous and find it difficult to eat. Opioids, of course, work wonders for people in severe pain. Methamphetamines can be helpful when you need to keep awake. Perhaps truck drivers should not use them. However, they can be a blessing to soldiers at war. Even cocaine can be an effective local anesthetic. A few studies show that nicotine can improve one's concentration. There is growing evidence that nicotine can be useful for Parkinson's disease.

I was at the University of Texas in the 1960's. Marijuana was everywhere; at parties, at concerts and at "happenings" (a gathering for no special purpose). I smoked it both for its effects and to fit in with my friends. I believe that marijuana made the Beetle's movie "Yellow

Submarine" an exceptional experience. I was in no danger of becoming addicted for at least the following two reasons. One, I did not smoke cigarettes. Two, I never used it unless I was part of a group. On the other hand, I had close friends who also took LSD. One friend found LSD to be quite enlightening. Unfortunately, another friend ran down the street half-naked after taking it. Instead of using LSD myself, I talked down people at a drop-in center who were having a bad trip.

As I mentioned earlier, my father was an alcoholic. I drink alcohol very sparingly. In some ways it seems like a contradiction that the children of alcoholics are more likely to become one themselves. I don't think the primary reason is genetics. I believe it is because adolescents of alcoholics have easy access to alcohol, they can be popular by supplying their friends with alcohol, and their parents are probably not the best at monitoring their children's behaviors.

I also believe that one of the problems with most books on the opioid crisis is that they ignore the opioid users who are not addicted. This is particularly true when it comes to a neurological explanation of addiction. These explanations clearly show how someone becomes addicted but do not explain how it is possible for some people to use opioids and not become addicted.

Let me give you an example regarding alcohol. For years people were taught that alcohol dehydrates you. I went to a seminar where the group decided we should not choose a carton of beer to help us survive in the desert because alcohol dehydrates you. Having worked with alcoholics and studied how the body digests alcohol, I objected. I said that although water would be better than alcohol, our bodies break down alcohol into carbon dioxide and water. I was voted down!

After retirement, I would occasionally join three other retirees under a raised house where we would drink beer. Whereas my limit was two beers, the others drank several. Even though there was a downstairs toilet 20 feet from where we drank, I do not remember any of the heavy beer drinking using it. How is that possible if alcohol dehydrates you?

As it turns out, the explanation is provided by neuroscientist Judith Grisel. She says the following three laws apply to all drugs (*Never Enough*, p. 30):

> (1) All drugs act by changing the rate of what is already going on.
>
> (2) All drugs have side effect.
>
> (3) The brain adapts to all drugs that affect it by counteracting the drug's effects.

Law number 3 relates to homeostasis (i.e., maintaining stability). With respect to the beer drinkers, a little alcohol might dehydrate you but a lot of alcohol has the opposite effect. An educated guess of mine is that if you are dying of thirst in the desert, your body is smart enough to retain water formed from breaking down alcohol.

Heavy use of opioids causes your body to counteract the effects of the drugs by creating tolerance.

In other words, you will need to up your dose to get the "high" you desire. I therefore conclude that a person could take opioids in moderation if their episodes were far enough apart to prevent tolerance. Evidently, the ancient Greeks were on to something when they said "Everything in moderation." (Note: I am not advocating opioid use in moderation.) We all know that nicotine is highly addictive and yet there are many smokers who are able to limit the number of cigarettes smoked. Clearly, we need more research on people who take addictive substances and do not become addicted.

As to the dehydrating effects of alcohol, "An Institute of Medicine (IOM) expert panel concluded that most Americans get plenty of water not only from plain water but also from food, milk, juice, and even coffee, tea, and alcoholic beverages" (*Tufts Health & Nutrition Letter*, June 2017).

Cultural Considerations

The use of opioids and other illicit drugs has gone up over the last ten plus years. I do not know the solution but I know what is not the solution. Better addiction treatment is not the solution. More drug prevention classes in the schools is not the solution. In all probability the solution will involve cultural changes.

As I mentioned earlier, Union soldiers were given opium but we do not have a good handle on how many became addicted. We also know that morphine was commonly given years ago to hospital patients as a pain killer and very few people became addicted.

We have recently begun a cultural solution to reducing opioid dependence by encouraging fewer prescriptions of opioids for pain and more closely monitoring those who need them. A review of 67 studies on tapering opioids for pain patients found only 3 to be of "high quality" (Krebs et al, reported in *Scientific American*, Oct. 2018). This same review recommended "very close patient follow-up." In another study of 68 chronic pain patients, 51 of those patients cut their opioid dosage nearly in half in four months without increased pain (ibid). A study reported in *JAMA* (March, 2018) concluded that "Results do not support initiation of opioid therapy for moderate to severe chronic back pain or hip or knee osteoarthritic pain." A review of 21 studies found that Cognitive Behavioral Therapy (CBT) and Mindfulness-Based-Stress Reduction (MBSR) were able to reduce pain (*Evidence-Based Mental Health*, Jan. 31, 2019).

Some of the alternate ways of treating pain include methods of relaxation, physical therapy, acupuncture, massage, heat, and electrical nerve stimulation. Non-opioid medications for pain include antidepressants, tranquilizers, anticonvulsants, and antiarrhythmics.

"Of all who tried any narcotic in Vietnam, 79 percent used heroin, as did 74 percent of those who took any narcotic since Vietnam. But the overall rate of narcotic use in the months since return from Vietnam had changed very little from the rate reported for men before leaving for Vietnam.' ... There have been no studies of addict populations in this country that show anything like the 95 percent remission rate after ten months, which is what a drop from 20 percent addicted while in Vietnam to 1 percent after Vietnam suggests. On the other hand, there has never been a situation in this country in which addicts make up 20 percent of a general population" (Robins et al, Washington University School of Medicine, grant, 1974).

Are there cultural/sociological differences that help explain the varying rates of addiction? Neurologist Carl Hart was raised in a poor black neighborhood. He believes that a strong negative bias exists toward drug use because the studies are funded by the National Institute of Drug Abuse. ("*High Price*" published by Harper in 2014)

I once ran a stop smoking program (volunteer work). Which statement would get me the most clients?

(A) I can double your chances of quitting smoking with my program, or

(B) I have a success rate of 25%. (I actually had 2 of 7 quit = 29%.)

Both of the above statements are true. The success rate for quitting smoking is about 12%. Whereas there is money to be had by doubling your chances of quitting an opioid with treatment, no one wants to pay money to improve their odds of going without nicotine to 25%. Even popular medications to help stop smoking (varenicline and bupropion) had at best a 20% success rate. Furthermore, Varenicline (Chantix) has some potential serious side effects including suicidal thoughts and heart problems.

The importance of cultural considerations is important when you consider the addiction to nicotine, otherwise known as smoking. About 50 years ago, 42% of

U.S. adults smoked. In 2005, 20.9 percent smoked and that dropped to 15.5% in 2016 (about 38 million Americans) according to the Centers for Disease Control and Prevention.

Clearly, the reduction in smoking in the United States had nothing to do with treatment and very little to do with education. The following steps helped:

(1) Taxed cigarettes
(2) Sued manufacturers (false statements)
(3) Made cigarettes come with a warning
(4) Restricted the use of cigarette advertisements
(5) Banned cigarettes in restaurants, public places, work places, etc.
(6) Launched propaganda programs
(7) Educated children
(8) Created E-cigarettes

Probably the most underrated action we took was we rarely show people smoking in the movies and on television (Unless you watch Turner Classics). We could use the above methods to reduce the use of heroin but we would first have to make it legal!

Another cultural phenomenon is our prejudice against old people. Ten times more people die from smoking than from opioids. Those who smoke heavily die as much as ten years early. Furthermore, twice as many people die per year from alcohol abuse than opioids. I believe that we especially care about opioid deaths because they kill young people.

Almost 4% of all deaths worldwide are attributed to alcohol (Global status report on alcohol and health, World Health Organization 2011). "A recent analysis of 112 studies on the effects of alcohol tax increases affirmed that when taxes go up, drinking goes down, including among problem drinkers and youth" (Ibid). Instead of paying schools for drug and alcohol prevention programs, we could be making money and reducing problem drinking at the same time! Taxing sugary soft drinks could do the same for type 2 diabetes.

Based on a 2015 Survey of 15- and 16-year-olds in 35 European countries (European School Survey Project on Alcohol and Other Drugs (ESPAD), daily smoking in the United States was 3% and 12% in Europe. On the other hand, 35% of the US sample had used an illicit drug compared to 18% of the European teens.

It is well documented that most Europeans drink more alcohol than people in the United States. Less clear is whether we differ in the percent of drinkers who have problems (i.e., become alcoholics). According to the World Health Organization referred to above, people in the United States engage in more "risky" drinking than Europeans. Drinking with meals would be an example of low risk drinking.

We saw what happened in Switzerland in the 1990's when they administered free heroin. HIV went down 50%. "Drug-related deaths under the age of 35 fell from 305 in 1995 to 25 in 2015. ... Crime linked to heroin has almost disappeared" (*The Nation*, Internet, Nov. 9,

2018). We in the United States believe in punishment, not statistics.

Portugal has decriminalized most street drugs and their social problems did not increase. HIV infection plummeted from an all-time high in 2000 of 104.2 new cases per million to 4.2 cases per million in 2015. As of 2012, Portugal's drug death toll was 3 per million, in comparison to the EU average of 17.3 per million.

Vancouver, Canada has a program where addicts can take heroin in a safe environment with clean needles. In 14 years, no one has died of a drug overdose at Insite or any other supervised injection site in Vancouver (bbc.com, Aug. 7, 2017 Internet).

In 2008, The Brookings Institute compared our model of punishing/imprisoning drug addicts to the more lenient policies in Europe. Our correctional approach has been a failure. The United States user rate for hard drugs that is about four times higher than Europe.

The Cato Institute (July 23, 2018) estimates that "drug legalization could generate up to $106.7 billion in annual budgetary gains for federal, state, and local governments. Those gains would come from two primary sources: decreases in drug enforcement spending and increases in tax revenue. This bulletin estimates that state and local governments spend $29 billion on drug prohibition annually, while the federal government spends an additional $18 billion. Meanwhile, full drug legalization would yield $19 billion in state and local tax revenue and

$39 billion in federal tax revenue." Drug legalization would create all the money needed for my system of referral and follow-up and still have some monies for addiction treatment and prevention.

The FY2018 Drug Control budget requested a little over 5 billion dollars for interdiction. I assume this means trying to keep illegal drugs from entering this country. Does our government attempt to bring illegal drugs into this country to test what percent make it in successfully? I have read that we intercept only 10% of illegal drugs entering this country but I do not know the source of that information. How many illegal drugs do we intercept coming in from Canada? Interdiction seems like a poor use of money. I suggest we randomly search people, vessels and vehicles with considerably less money and that we do not publish these figures. When the news media reports a huge drug bust do you consider that good news or bad news?

A popular strategy of law enforcement is to go after drug dealers. One problem with this approach is that users often become small time dealers to support their habit. However, the biggest problem with going after dealers, in my opinion, is that there is so much money in drugs that others soon take their place. The *Times Picayune* (2014) reported two drug dealers found guilty of racketeering. According to the District Attorney, they were turning a profit of $400,000 monthly. If this is true, not only is going after dealers a bad solution but it is counterproductive. On the other hand, I have never heard of someone say they took up drugs because they know of a user that had gone to jail.

We would have dealt with our opioid problem earlier if it were not for the power of our largest lobby – the pharmaceutical industry. Within the last ten years, OxyContin was bringing in $1.5 billion per year, a pain clinic in West Virginia was taking in $20,000 per day in cash, over 250 million opioid prescription per year were written and three-fourths of accidental drug overdoses were prescription drugs (Chris McGreal, *American Overdose*, 2018).

Would decriminalization work in the United States? Drug courts represent a cultural change. Drug courts have allowed more people to be diverted away from prison and into treatment. Marijuana is now legal in some states. (Technically, the Federal Government says it is still illegal.) Gambling is an official addiction although it is legal in some form in all but two states (Hawaii and Utah).

Thomas and Margulis (*The Addiction Spectrum*, 2018) say that addiction is a public-health crisis. I agree. We need to make drastic changes, not more of the same. We could quickly make inroads to the damage heroin does by providing free heroin in closely monitored clinics. These same clinics would not only encourage users to get clean but would provide free opioid agonists and antagonists and monitor their use. We already have data to show that making medical marijuana legal did not increase the use of marijuana among teens. In California, the number of pot smoking teenagers went down after medical marijuana became legal in 1996. Other states that followed showed no change in teenage use (*Live Science*, Feb. 22, 2018 Internet).

We also have data that indicates that lowering the drinking age in the 1970's led to increased drinking in adolescents and more auto fatalities. We know that taxing cigarettes and alcohol reduces consumption although taxes mostly affect moderate users.

Books written on addiction seem quick to recommend something based on research and slow to recommend something that works in the real world. They mention the liberal drug policies of Portugal, the Netherlands, Switzerland and Canada as something to "think about". I don't have to think about it. Neither does Ryan Hampton (*American Fix*). I would rather spend $30,000 on a clinic that provided free heroin in a safe and monitored environment than spend the money for the treatment of a single client who will still have only a 50% chance of not relapsing.

Buying heroin on the street has at least four problems. One, the heroin might not be pure. Two, the buyer might need medical assistance. Three, the buyer might get arrested. Four, buying drugs on the street supports a thriving criminal enterprise. Providing heroin in a clinic allows the staff to build rapport with someone who may later decide to accept help in getting clean.

Even with the recommendations from popular books on addiction, the influence of scholars appears to be rather weak. In 2006, William Miller and Kathleen Carroll edited a very scholarly and informative book titled

"*Rethinking Substance Abuse*. This book had input from 19 Ph.D.'s, 5 M.D.'s and 2 persons with bachelor degrees. I wonder how much this book has led to real world progress in the last 12 years.

Looking over the last 40 years, I have seen the remarkable drop in cigarette smoking. I see crack cocaine versus powder cocaine being rethought after sending a disproportionate number of black men to prison. I see more states legalizing medical marijuana as well as recreational marijuana. Sentences are being reduced for drug offenses and drug courts are diverting people to treatment. I can only conclude the following:
The greatest gains made in the United States regarding drug abuse have been made by lawyers and politicians!

Also, where drugs are not a commodity (bought and sold), few problems exist. Which is worse – the use of illegal drugs or the business of selling illegal drugs? Selling illegal drugs often leads to violence over territory and innocent people might be collateral damage. People who use drugs often end up being dealers to pay for their costs.

Cultures that use mind changing drugs as a ritual (i.e., peyote, ayahuasca, ibogaine) have few problems. Social parameters help. Starting your day with a cup of coffee is a ritual. So is taking a smoking break at work. Toasting the bride and groom is a ritual. So is taking communion at church. In my day, passing a joint (marijuana) around at a concert was a ritual. Unfortunately, using alcohol are part of a hazing in a college fraternity has had unfavorable results.

Native Americans have the highest incidence of heavy drinking (12.1%) of our various ethnic groups (National Survey on Drug Use and Health, SAMHSA 2008). "Teens on Native American reservations continue to be more likely to report using alcohol, marijuana and other illicit drugs than peers elsewhere in the U.S. and to start using at younger ages." (*Health News*, June 7, 2018). Government officials have been working with Native American reservations for decades on these problems with no resolution in sight. Clearly this calls for a cultural solution led by Native American community leaders.

Does a 57% relapse rate for one year with 40% occurring in the first 6 months sound like drug addiction? This is the recidivism rate for people leaving state prisons, the closest analogy I could find to drug abuse. Many people believe it is the nature of drug addicts to have a high relapse just as it is the nature of criminals to be repeat offenders. So how do we explain that the recidivism rate from federal prisons is 45% over five years versus 77% for state prisons? Norway imprisons one-tenth fewer people per populations than the United States. The recidivism rate for Norway is 20%. We may never be another Norway but I do not accept a prison recidivism rate of 57% as reasonable any more than I accept an addiction relapse rate of 57% as reasonable.

Just as the United States will never be another Norway, will Louisiana ever be a Minnesota? Both states are similar in population and similar in the distribution of population among large cites, small towns and rural areas. When I did a crime comparison several years ago (1990, *Uniform Crime Reports*), I discovered that the murder rate in Louisiana was <u>over six times</u> that of Minnesota. Even within Louisiana, the chance of getting murdered in a large city is nearly double that of living in a small town. In all fairness, I believe there is a geographical effect. It is difficult to commit a crime in below zero-degree weather. There are a lot of ways to improve your safety but have you thought of moving?

I predict that you will soon be seeing statistics from states that have legalized marijuana as to incidents of increased psychological and medical problems. A European study found that daily users of high potency (THC > 10%) marijuana were more than four times more likely to be given a first-time diagnosis of psychosis than non-users (*The Lancet*, March 19, 2019). Users in Amsterdam users were twice as likely to become psychotic than users in Paris. About 1% of the world population are psychotic (mostly schizophrenic). Marijuana varies greatly in THC levels much like alcoholic beverages vary in percent alcohol. Similar to alcohol, only adults should use marijuana and they should use it in moderation. Keep in mind that the problems with marijuana might be preferable to the problems and costs of incarcerating people for drug offenses. Hard to evaluate are the costs of trying to get a job after coming from prison. Again, most people do not think in terms of systems. Some people are interested in addiction and some people are interested in corrections and few realize that they have to be considered together. Of course, one reason for legalizing marijuana was that it was considered to be no worse than alcohol or cigarettes. Will new evidence change this? Marijuana is being cultivated with higher levels of THC. Unlike opioids, THC acts throughout the brain (*Never Enough*, p.55).

I am all for drug courts, diversion programs, and reducing the sentencing for drug offenses. However, people who advocate for these changes are probably missing the big picture. **The big picture is that we are one of the most punitive countries on the planet!** If our correctional system was more like Norway or Germany, we would not have to divert anyone.

The United States has a Surgeon General. Perhaps we need a Sociologist General to brief Congress on what other nations do for controlling health costs, reducing prison recidivism, creating equality, and reducing substance abuse. The 1958 book *"The Ugly American"* portrayed the arrogance and insensitivity of Americans who visited other countries. Even today, politicians are quick to point out the countries we do not want to emulate. When have you ever heard a politician mention a country we want to be more like? Do we want a government with less corruption like New Zealand? Do we want a country where students excel in academics like Finland? Do we want good health care like Switzerland? Evidently not, according to our politicians.

Is drug addiction a medical problem, psychological problem or both? If the opioid crisis is considered an epidemic, then why aren't epidemiologists, sociologists, and anthropologists in charge? A group of people led by Georgiy Bobashev created a model called "Pain Town" ("Model Citizens", *Scientific American*, Special Edition, Winter 2018/2019.). This is a city with 10,000 people suffering from chronic pain complete with 30 doctors, 10 emergency rooms, 10 pharmacies and 70 drug dealers. They run this model over five years as drug tolerances increase, doctors write prescriptions, drug dealers need increased supplies and overdoses increase. Early data suggests that requiring physicians to track medication histories can be effective in the long term. Models have the capability of being expanded, tested and refined. Variables, such as arrests, can be modeled to look at long term effects. The University of Pittsburgh has a model called a Framework for Reconstructing Epidemiological Dynamics (FRED). It is going to model opioid use based on historical trends.

Which solutions work the best? You saw the example with cigarettes. The best approach was clearly cultural. So, what are some cultural solutions for drug abuse?

We have recently made changes in prescribing opioids for pain. Prescriptions are more time limited and smaller doses are prescribed. Still, we do not want to exacerbate the pain of people with serious medical problems. Some of the nonmedical approaches to pain management include massage, yoga, meditation and exercise. Some people believe acupuncture is also effective for reducing pain. A 2012 study of 240 veterans who suffered from persistent pain were assigned to either an opioid group or a nonopioid group. "Patients given alternative drugs did just as well as those taking opioids in terms of how much pain interfered with their everyday life" (*Scientific American*, June 2018).

For preventing drug abuse, I would rather put money into teen "nightclubs" over school prevention programs. Teens need a place, other than the mall, where they can hangout with minimal opportunities for trouble. Perhaps we need a "Chuckie Cheese" for teens; a place where they can have fun without drugs or alcohol. Although it is possible that a commercial place such as one with laser tag or video games can succeed, I believe we need tax sponsored places where even teens without money can go and have fun.

Several years ago, New Orleans tried midnight basketball. Middle class people from intact families thought the idea was ridiculous. I thought that midnight basketball for young males from the inner city was much preferred over taking drugs and petty theft. According to the Town of Manchester, Connecticut website "Juvenile criminal activity dropped 24% in Cincinnati, Ohio during the first 13 weeks of their late-night basketball program. Summer late night weekend recreation activities costing only 74 cents per person reduced juvenile crime by 52% in Phoenix, Arizona where it costs almost $40,000 to jail one teen for one year. The bottom line is it costs 100 times as much to incarcerate than to recreate."

People in abstinence-contingent housing with recreational activities and skill-building courses were more successful (50% abstinence) than those with just Contingency Management (37%) or traditional treatment

(13%) (Rash et al, *Journal of Substance Abuse Treatment*, Jan. 2017, Vol. 72).

Many addiction treatment facilities have art (37%) and music (15%) therapy available (Based on a sample from 299 treatment facilities who responded out of 451). I could not find any data if these activities reduce relapse rates. It is known that music has been helpful with stroke patients and persons with autism. Brain imaging studies show that "making music spur activity and foster connections across a wide swath of brain regions typically involved in emotion, reward, cognition, sensation and movement" (*Scientific American Mind*, March/April, 2015). Evidently, music hijacks the brain.

Recently, several colleges have created drug and alcohol-free dorms. Students sign a pledge who choose to live in one of these dorms. These dorms do their best to provide for healthy activities such as exercise, yoga, meditation and even healthy nutrition options. Colleges should provide free mentoring, classes on improving study habits and other general topics of interest to dorm students. Furthermore, they should provide something extra to the alcohol-free/drug-free dorms that no one else gets such as free concert tickets.

Whereas the differences in treatment methods are small, the differences in cultures are large. Remember that Ireland's study on opioid relapse was 91% and the relapse rate of India's study was 32%. In Ghana, the relapse rate is 75% within the first 6 months (Appiah et al, *Journal of Drug Issues*, 2017, 47(1)). Ghana is a poor country where it is considered impolite to refuse an alcoholic drink.

The percent of smokers in the United States went from 42% of the populations to 15.5% as the result of cultural changes whereas the relapse rate appears to be unchanged. There is even a rat study done in the 1970's that demonstrated that rats given an enriched environment preferred water over morphine (Alexander, *Psychopharmacology*, 1978 (58)). (Note: This study might be dependent on the strain of rats used.)

One possible reason for so little interest in cultural change is to look at who is in charge of addiction programs and funding. The National Institute of Drug Abuse has an editorial staff of 17 persons. Are any of these people sociologists or anthropologists? What are the qualifications of the people who are in charge of addiction for the states?

Another possible reason for so little interest in culture is that so many books are written by former addicts and alcoholics. They say a fish has no concept of water. How many of these authors have lived in other parts of the world? As previously mentioned, cultures that use drugs as part of rituals and not as a marketable commodity have few problems.

Does anyone believe that high schools teaching young boys the value of respecting women could match the gains achieved by the "MeToo" movement? The influence of cultural changes far exceeds education and counseling. How about getting *Facebook* to launch a massive campaign showing people who use drugs as losers? At the time of this writing, *Facebook* is facing problems of integrity. Wouldn't they want to be a part of a program to prevent substance abuse? The influence of M.D.'s and Ph.D.'s is diminishing. What we need is a Justin Bieber or some other popular young person to take on drug abuse. **I believe that any major shift in the use of drugs in the United States will be created by young people.**

We already know that every group a person belongs to can be a support group, not just AA and NA. Being married or in a significant relationship can reduce the impact of genetics favoring addiction. Of course, groups can work in the opposite direction when peers use their influence to coerce others to emulate their anti-social behaviors. It is known that when observing a group of drinkers, it is the heaviest drinkers that set the pace.

I have one cultural solution for our drug crisis – make it illegal for pharmaceutical companies to give physicians anything free with the exception of samples. Martin Schram (*Tribune News Service*) says that according to a study done by the Boston Medical Center and New York University School of Medicine, there were more opioid overdose deaths in countries where physicians received the most money from pharmaceutical companies. "Opioid manufacturers spent about $40 million on meals, trips and consulting fees for almost 68,000 doctors from 2013 through 2015". In other words, let's have no more free lunches, wall decorations, trips or paid conferences. Any medical conference of any value should be sponsored by the United States government or hospitals, not pharmaceutical companies. Of course, these same restrictions would have to apply to politicians.

The pharmaceutical industry is the largest lobby in the United States spending about $250 million per year. The top four pharmaceutical companies make over $25 billion per year. In 2019, Purdue Pharma, maker of OxyContin, agreed to pay $270 million of which $200 million will establish the National Center for Addiction Studies and Treatment. Furthermore, "Federal prosecutors charged drug distributor Rochester Drug Cooperative and its former CEO with drug trafficking charges Tuesday -- the first criminal charges for a pharmaceutical company and executives in the nation's ongoing opioid crisis" (ABC News, April 23, 2019). From 2012 to 2016, RDC's sales of oxycodone tablets grew 800 percent and its fentanyl sales grew 2000 percent.

Although pharmaceutical companies have paid out millions in law suits, this did not stop them from coming out with an opioid (Dsuvia) stronger than fentanyl.

Perhaps suing the Food and Drug Administration (FDA) is a better idea.

Congress is looking for ways to lower drug costs. They are looking at the patent process, group/government purchases, and why medications are cheaper in other countries.

I have another cultural solution for drug abuse. It is based on my experience with restaurants. Have you ever gotten food poisoning from a restaurant? I have. I felt like I was going to die. Fortunately, it was over in 24 hours. Guess what? I never returned to that restaurant! It only took <u>one episode</u> to change my mind about a restaurant I had enjoyed several times in the past. This is an effective method because evolution dictates that avoiding death takes precedence over the greatest of pleasures. Of course, the person has to be aware of impending death.

Law enforcement seizes a lot of illegal drugs. They also infiltrate the organizations of drug dealers to gather evidence and make arrests. I suggest that instead of making arrests, they surreptitiously sell back drugs that have been tainted to make people sick (but not die) to other drug dealers. Antabuse works like this for people who drink alcohol. Of course, only a small fraction of these drugs needs to be tainted to make it difficult to discover from where the drugs came. Over time, most drug users would eventually hit a tainted batch. Of course, it may take more than one episode for a seasoned user to want to change.

This approach would work best if our government provided our addicts with drugs known to be clean. Switzerland, the Netherlands, and Portugal already provide this service. In 2017, Norway became the first Scandinavian county to decriminalize drugs. In 2020, Norway expects to provide drug users with free heroin.

Many psychologists have done a great disservice by convincing the public that punishment does not work. If you ever want to housebreak a puppy, you follow him around with a rolled-up newspaper and when it appears he is about to go on your carpet you swat him with the newspaper and then put him outdoors. Psychologists would have you believe that you will have to follow your dog around with a rolled-up newspaper the rest of his life. Punishment works when it is immediate. If you have ever poured water on a pan full of grease while learning how to cook, you will only do it once. Unfortunately, by the time a man goes to prison for a drug offense, he has convinced himself it is because of his skin color or for a victimless crime or because society favors some drugs (i.e., alcohol) over others.

My opinion on the "War on Drugs" as printed in the *Times Picayune* in 1989 is given in Appendix 6.

I believe that replacing physicians and psychologists in charge of addiction at the governmental level with statisticians and sociologists would be a good idea. Even better would be to put persons with Masters in Business Administration (MBA's) in charge of everything. This idea is based on the concept that management is its own specialty. I believe that very few experts would choose to be managers if it involved a reduction in pay. This is a radical cultural change which would finally get rid of "The Peter Principle"; that people get promoted until they reach their level of incompetence.

Dr. Deming taught me "Don't change people, change the system." Fewer accidents occur on the road because of the following safety improvements – collision warning, automatic braking, lane departure warning, pedestrian detection, adaptive cruise control, blind spot warning, rear traffic alert and road sign recognition.

I suggest we add driver impairment recognition as a standard safety feature. In other words, when you first turn on your vehicle you would have to respond to instructions on the screen to show you can make appropriate quick decisions. You would get two tries to get it right. Failure would mean that you cannot start your vehicle for an hour. What about emergencies? You would have an emergency button. However, when you press it, the police would be informed. A police office will not take well to an emergency button pressed by someone under the influence of alcohol or another drug. Of course, it would be against the law for someone other than the driver to do the driver impairment test. You could even have approved thumb prints for persons authorized to drive a certain vehicle.

One recent cultural change is the increased use of Uber. I expect Uber will keep fewer impaired people from driving. At least one study backs this up. "It found that in four boroughs of New York City, excluding Staten Island, there has been a 25 to 35 percent reduction in alcohol-related car accidents since Uber came to town in 2011, as compared to other places where a ride-hailing company doesn't operate" (nytimes.com/2017/04/07). During New Year's Eve, the local police in New Orleans offer free rides to prevent accidents. We need a year-round service such as this for persons under the influence of alcohol, drugs or medication.

Another simple idea is to give all movies that portray drug use as "fun" be given an 'R' rating. Movies that show the dangers and tragedies of drug use would be rated 'PG 13'.

Just as we have suicide hot lines, we need many hot lines for substance abuse. These people can help calm people down and provide information and other local sources of assistance. Presently, SAMSHA has a national help line that is always open (1-800-662-HELP). There are also at least six youth friendly online resources.

We need more than help over the telephone and Internet. Every city should have a free place where people high on drugs can go to for assistance. These facilities, staffed by medical personnel, would be similar to an urgent care facility. However, they would be funded by public monies and persons using such a facility could remain anonymous. Great Falls has a drop-in center for addiction. Persons in Hudson/Marlborough have a drop-in center for substance abuse. Don't be fooled. Many drop-in centers are affiliated with treatment centers. I have no idea how many of these places allow people to remain anonymous. I only know that I volunteered at a drop-in center in the 1960's that met the above criteria.

Milieu

In Minnesota I chaired a two-day conference on program evaluation attended by people from all over the state. At the time I was interested in creating a measure of the milieu of psychiatric and addiction treatment centers. Milieu is essentially the culture of a limited surrounding. Milieu is a reflection of how an individual in an addiction center is treated. Does the staff show compassion? Do they respect your opinion? Can you choose the treatment methods you think will work? Will they discharge you when you think you are ready? Are visiting hours reasonable? Of course, some of the amenities of a treatment facility depends on how much it costs. A treatment center's philosophy is also a part of the milieu. Let me describe some stereotypes.

"Authoritarian" describes the medical model. If some of the people in a treatment center go by the title "doctor", the philosophy is at least, in part, authoritarian. In an authoritarian setting, people with degrees tell you what you need to do. "You need to quit entirely." "You need to learn to relax." "You need to take medicine such as an opioid agonist." Think of the last time you were given a prescription. Did the physician ask if you intended to use it? Physicians know a lot more about medicine than I do. On the other hand, my car mechanic knows a lot more about cars than I do. When I have my car repaired, the waiting room has free coffee and donuts plus a giant television. When I visit my physician, I sit in a room full of old magazines.

"True Believers" is my name for another type of treatment philosophy. No priest is ever going to tell you "I think you would do better with Buddhism." In my day, Alcoholics Anonymous was a true believer. Based on their advertisements, a local treatment center that uses a nutritional approach sounds like a true believer. If you are in a treatment center run by former addicts/alcoholics, there is a good chance they are true believers.

"Client-Centered" is my name for treatment centers that revolve around Motivational Interviewing and Non-Directive Therapy. "Laissez-faire" reflects our feelings down in the "Big Easy". It pretty much means let everyone do what they feel they need to do. This is the exact opposite of the authoritarian method. The client is in charge. Clients choose their own goals and treatment methods. Should the family be involved? Do I need medications including opiate agonists? What new activities should I take up? The client needs to make a lot of decisions.

Taking client-centered to an extreme is what I call the "Pampered" philosophy. I believe Arizona has a few of these treatment centers - spa's with massage and whirlpools, walks in the sunshine, meditation and soft music. Throw in a few lectures and you are good to go.

"Empirical" would be my philosophy if I were running a treatment center. Lots of people would be running around measuring things. We would be not big believers in talk. We like to see target behaviors met. We would then work backwards to see what is the best way to create these behaviors. If this sounds academic and cold to you, I call it humble and realistic. Some treatment centers are full of testimonials. Some mention their staff of Ph.D.'s and M.D.'s. Other treatment centers pride themselves on using only evidence-based methods. Guess what? Treatment centers that refer to "state of the art" therapies are stagnant in my opinion. I would never use the term "state of the art" because I find a success rate of 50% to be embarrassing. I would want our clients to know that as they get better, we get better. We could call this approach results-centered. We would be equal partners, neither client centered nor authoritarian.

Remember that prescription you were given? Did someone call you a few days later to see how you were doing? Today a computer could email you a series of questions regarding your office visit. That computer could even take your responses and put them in a database and later create a report on everyone in a similar situation. Medicine is in the dark ages regarding the power of data mining. First, we need a universal medical record that all physicians can use. Second, we need to figure out how to maintain each person's privacy. Of course, there would still be the problem of non-responders. However, an asthmatic is less likely to blame himself for an ineffective treatment than someone receiving counseling, going to meetings, or taking suboxone for an addiction to heroin.

Control Groups

I believe that most people have misconceptions regarding the placebo effect. Let's start with "New Age" thinking. New Age thinking is best summarized in the following saying: "If the mind can conceive it, and truly believe it, you can achieve it."

One of the most popular self-help books ever written was called "The Power of Positive Thinking" by Norman Vincent Peale in 1952. This book sold over 15 million copies and was translated into over 40 languages.

In the 1920's Emile Coue created the mantra "Every day, in every way, I'm getting better and better".

He believed that if you could completely occupy the mind with an idea it would become a reality.

Long before either of the above, Jesus said "Truly I tell you, if you have faith as small as a mustard seed, you can say to this mountain, 'Move from here to there,' and it will move. Nothing will be impossible for you" (Mathew 17:20).

The placebo is anything that will change one's thinking to either

(A) create an outcome in line with one's expectations or
(B) lead the person to believe that such an outcome has already taken place.

Consequently, every time you see a physician or a therapist, the placebo effect is operating. Every legitimate treatment involves the placebo effect.

In many cases, the placebo effect is larger than the specific effect of the treatment. Consider the following study done in 2008 (*British Medical Journal*, May) on Irritable Bowel Syndrome. Of persons in the no treatment group, 28% felt relief. Of those given fake acupuncture, 44% felt relief. For those given fake acupuncture by a warm, empathetic doctor, 62% felt relief.

Not all control groups are alike. Many drug studies over the years have shown the power of the placebo. In general, about 30% of improvement from any medical or psychological treatment can be attributed to the placebo effect. Not only are placebos powerful but two placebos work better than one, and a placebo that tastes awful or produces side effects works even better. As popular as antidepressants are, fifteen major reviews of the literature found that 30 to 40 percent of the studies show no significant difference in response to drug versus placebo (Fisher and Greenberg, *Psychology Today*, Sep./Oct. 1995). Another review of antidepressant drug studies found that drugs reduced depressive symptoms by 41% whereas placebos reduced depressive symptoms 31% (Warner and Brown, "Symptom Reduction and Suicide risk in Patients Treatment with Placebo in Antidepressant Clinical Trials," (*Archives of General Psychiatry*, 2000 (57)). A meta-analysis of placebo-controlled studies of antidepressants by Kirsch et al found that 80% of the positive response to these medications might be the placebo effect (*Harvard Mental Health Letter*, Mar. 2003). Keep in mind that studies that show no differences are less likely to be reported than studies that show promising treatment effects. Placebos are powerful. They can produce "toxic effects such as rashes, apparent memory loss, fever, headaches, and more" (*ibid.*).

A person's expectations are so important that in one study, subjects who were injected with salt water thought to be allergenic got symptoms of itching, burning, and nausea. Upon given the same injection of salt water said to be a "neutralizing" injection they got better (*Sickness and Healing: An Anthropological Perspective*, Robert Hahn, 1995). Another study found that giving cancer patients a placebo lead to nausea in one-third of the patients, vomiting in one-fifth, while almost one-third lost hair (*Psychology Today*, March/April, 1997). Just as placebos thought to be medications help people improve, a small number of studies have shown that medications thought to be placebos are less effective. Furthermore, double-blind studies have to be questioned if the placebo does not produce any effects at all. Physical reactions (i.e., side effects) help patients believe the medication is really working.

The American Medical Association looked at 96 studies involving 26,00 patients living with chronic noncancer pain. This research "suggests that prescription opioids may offer little more benefit than placebos for patients who are being treated for long-term noncancer-related pain" (*Times Picayune*, Dec.23, 2018). Interestingly, the placebo effect probably involves the production of endogenous opioids given that Naloxone reduces the placebo effect (Grevert et al, *Pain*, 1983, Jun. 16(2)).

Recent studies using techniques such as positron emission tomography (PET) and quantitative electroencephalography (QEEG) have demonstrated brain responses to placebos. Interestingly, the brain responses to placebos do not mimic the brain responses to antidepressants but differ from the non-responses of controls who receive neither (*Harvard Mental Health Letter*, Mar. 2003).

One might conceptualize the concept of the placebo as common factors involved with most types of treatment. Thus, common factors might include the expectation for improvement, therapist confidence, and a warm, understanding and accepting therapist. Even when we deal with a specific method such as cognitive therapy, it is possible that rewarding a specific behavior (contingency management) results in a cognitive change and vice-versa.

Fisher and Greenberg report "The literature is surprisingly full of instances of how social and attitudinal factors modify the effects of active drugs." For example, "Antipsychotic medications are more effective if the patient likes rather than dislikes the physician administering them." A study of vitamin E and another study of the drug meprobamate found the vitamin or drug to work only for the physicians who believed in it (*Healing Words* by Larry Dossey, p.135).

Most control groups for studies on the effectiveness of counseling or other psychological treatment use a group of people who are not given any treatment. For ethical reasons, sometime their treatment is "delayed." As I am a big believer in the power of placebos, I would like to see control groups assigned to fabricated treatments with scientific sounding theories. It is all too easy to beat a group of people who are told they are not receiving therapy. Bowers and Clum recommend studies should be controlled for (a) subject expectancy, (b) therapist expectancy, (c) placebo credibility, and (d) measurement reactivity. They also suggest that a placebo should involve the "interaction with a credentialed professional lasting as long as the specific treatment being assessed" ("Relative Contributions of Specific and Nonspecific Treatment Effects", *Psychological Bulletin*, 1988, vol. 103, p.315). In other words, a legitimate placebo for counseling would be to give the control group a treatment over a period of time that sounds scientific but has no real reason for working.

Just as the medical model is inappropriate for most psychological treatment, so the agricultural model of research based on applying different treatments to four fields of grain is not well suited for measuring the effectiveness of treatment. For example, people in the "no treatment" group might respond in a variety of different ways during the testing period. Some people might take a pro-active self-treatment approach; others rely on the support and advice of friends and family, while still others vegetate.

Fortunately, research into therapy is becoming more sophisticated. Hope Conte describes "The Evolving Nature of Psychotherapy Outcome Research" in the *American Journal of Psychotherapy,* 2001. She refers to the 1970's as a time when psychotherapy studies applied greater controls by sticking more closely to the scientific model of random assignments to well defined procedures. In the 1980' and 1990's more studies were done in natural clinical settings outside of universities. A strict reliance on official diagnostic criteria (i.e., DSM, primarily Axis I) were referred to as "research clinical trials". Conte refers to Beutler and his colleagues who say "Multiple patient dimensions, therapist dimensions, and therapy attributes must be incorporated into single analyses to assess the interchange among variables and their complex interactions in disposing patients to change."

Treatment centers for alcohol and drug addiction typically follow an "evidenced-based" program. Even

Louisiana's legislative report of 2017 begins with "THE OPIOID EPIDEMIC: EVIDENCE-BASED STRATEGIES". In other words, they use treatment approaches that studies have shown to be effective. These include the following therapies: Cognitive, behavioral, motivation interviewing, the Twelve Step program as well as pharmaceutical (Methadone, Buprenorphine).

The biggest problem with assessing the effectiveness of these programs is comparing them against suitable control groups. Comparing them against "no treatment" is not acceptable. As previously mentioned, placebos tend to outperform no treatment by as much as 30 percent.

The second major problem is controlling for patient motivation. Reporting the success rate for "persons who complete the program" or "persons who attend the most meetings" clearly does not control for a person's motivation.

In summary, the placebo effect convinces a person he can achieve success. A good counselor or friend does the same thing. Some therapists are able to maximize what I refer to as the "Shaman Effect". They use the power of their "Doctor" title along with a wall full of credentials. They assure their clients that they rely on "evidence based" methods. Consequently, it is a powerful technique when a respected therapist can convince a client that a treatment will work.

Many therapists have pointed out the inappropriateness of controlled experiments to test the effects of various treatments. George Silberschatz says "Our research clearly shows that effective therapists adapt their methods to the problems and needs of the individual patients. Close adherence to treatment manuals constrains this spontaneity, creativity, and flexibility" (*The Harvard Mental Health Letter*, July 1999).

I believe that evidence-based treatment can be relied on if an unbiased agency (the state?) collects standard outcome data from persons who were in actual treatment programs. In other words, the evidence is not based on university research. I requested the National Institute of Drug Abuse for a list of studies giving the relapse rates for inpatient addiction centers. I received a list of only two studies.

The first study was a longitudinal study of 4,229 persons from 76 addiction treatment programs including outpatient methadone treatment (OMT), Long-term residential treatment (LST) and outpatient drug free treatment (ODF). From Hubbard et al, *Journal of Substance Abuse Treatment*, 2003, 25(3).

For the OMT program, the one-year relapse rate was 26.5% and the five-year relapse rate was 34.2%. For LST the one-year relapse rate was 14.5% and the five-year relapse rate was 56.1 %. For ODF the one-year relapse rate was 50.6% and the five-year rate was 71.4%.

The first three figures seem remarkably low. The following facts make interpretation difficult. At year one, 70% of the original sample responded. However, that dropped to 33% at year five. The OMT group had about

50% more people over the age of 30 and about 70% more married persons, whereas the other two groups had 13 times as many persons who were referred by the criminal justice system.

Another table lists 75.2% persons using heroin at the one-year follow-up, 68.6% using heroin at the five-year follow-up, and 54.8% using heroin at both follow-ups (n=347). These figures are even higher than most studies.

The second study they referred me to lists relapse rates of 40% to 60% but does not give the details of a single study (McLellan et al, 2000, *JAMA* 284(13)).

Hazelden reported that a relapse rate of 47% (*Addictive Behaviors*, 1998, 23(5)). This was based on anonymous self-report of 767 of 1,083 clients (71%).

Why do so few studies of addiction treatment give a yearly relapse rate? I believe there are two reasons. One, people who do research do not want to wait a year before publishing their results. Two, the strength of their results could be greatly diminished a year later.

I like to see several sources of evidence before I get too enthused. As previously mentioned, I look first for meta-analysis studies. It is difficult, if not impossible, to find studies done by disinterested parties. Theories are fine for generating hypotheses but I think that some people are too quick to accept something with a good sounding explanation behind it (e.g., how the brain operates).

Statisticians use a method called "multiple regression" to make predictions. Typical of a multiple regression is that the first variable accounts for over 50% of the predictive power and as you add on other variables you get diminishing returns. In the case of addiction, you want to predict abstinence over a period of time based on the different treatment modalities. I would like to see more studies on addiction treatment use this regression model.

Try to find research that shows that addiction treatment centers that use five approaches do better than four or that four do better than three. Remember college? There is a point where adding too many credits to a semester begins to lower your grade point average. Without the appropriate follow-up research, I cannot say how many different approaches in one inpatient program really help. I previously mentioned one study that showed that adding contingency management got better results. I know that statisticians who do regression analysis typically find little predictive value beyond three or four variables. The only thing you can count on when treating the whole person is that it probably maximizes the placebo effect.

I believe that a combination of putting an addict in a healthy environment for 30 to 90 days along with the expectation of improvement (placebo effect) counts for over 50% of the benefits attributed to addiction treatment. Consequently, the following example of a treatment control group is necessary to gauge how much our various treatments actually contribute to an addict's improvement beyond this.

I am not aware of any studies that adequately compare an entire treatment program (see Appendix 7) against a suitable control group. Therefore, I am suggesting the following study.

Treatment Control Group

1. The Treatment Control Group (TCG) should last as many days as the Treatment Group (TG), usually 30, 60 or 90 days.
2. The TCG has no staff with advanced degrees and no certified addiction counselors or former addicts.
3. Persons in the TCG have a "normal" day consisting of breakfast, work, lunch, work, and dinner. (Note: Work is all in-house.)
4. Evenings are free time but they have available books, music, card tables and games (no computers, cell phones, electronic games or televisions are allowed as they can be an addiction). However, a regular line telephone will be available.
5. An exercise room is available as well as equipment for outdoor sports/activities.
6. A hiking trail and a nearby lake or pond would be ideal. (Note: The cheapest way to run this study would be to use a summer camp or religious retreat in the off-season.)
7. No free time activities are organized. Residents must show their own initiative.

8. Weekends are also free time. Sundays include a nondenominational religious service for those so inclined.
9. Friends and relatives are free to visit any time in the evenings or on weekends. (Note: This is not a cult.)

In summary, the TCG will have only three rules: You must work a normal 40-hour work week (or up to one's capacity), you cannot leave the grounds, and you will be expelled if you have any contraband including cell phones. Staff will only supervise work and prepare meals.

The TG and the TCG will be assessed primarily on relapse rates over given periods of time. Money received from the client's work (such as making something they can sell) will help pay the costs of the TCG.

Clients will not be told they are in a "control group". They will be told that they are in a program called "Normal Living." Clearly, living a normal life is not what addicts usually do.

Clearly this particular control group involves common factors. Subjects in typical treatment programs as well as this control group will believe they are in legitimate treatment. They will both spend several days without their addictive drugs and related behaviors. They will both spend a lot of time interacting with other sober/clean people. However, those person in addiction treatment centers will have a lot more structure. Those in the treatment control group will need to structure their own free time.

It is expected that those undergoing traditional treatment such as individual, group and family counseling as well as medically assisted treatment will produce more long-term gains than those in this control group. The question is "how much?" A key difference between the groups is that traditional treatment costs $10,000 per month and more whereas this control group will cost at most $1,000 per month depending on what products are produced during work time.

Cost is a major problem with addiction treatment. Insurance companies vary on their coverage of addiction treatment. I cannot blame them. Nearly everyone familiar with addiction treatment believe that some programs are bogus. A few might even be counterproductive. How can an insurance company separate the wheat from the chaff? Of course, my idea of creating a system of referral, treatment and follow-up would solve this problem.

The issue of paying for expensive illnesses needs to be addressed by the federal government. In France, the government covers all costs related to cancer treatment. With our aging population, our government will have to decide how to deal with Alzheimer's disease. Neither individuals or insurance companies have the resources for such a great expense. For those of you who believe the state has to provide addiction treatment for those who cannot afford it, perhaps they could run the "Normal Living" groups. Cost is certainly one of the reasons most addicts do not seek help. At less than $1,000 per month, a tremendous number of persons could now at least get minimal help.

Evidently, the experts in addiction do not agree with me as to the value of my Treatment Control Group. I submitted my idea to *The American Journal of Drug and Alcohol Abuse.* There response was "I regret to tell you that it has been decided not to process this manuscript through our review cycle. This decision is based on editorial considerations of the priority and relative importance of current submissions." The *Journal of Substance Abuse Treatment* replied "I feel that it is not suitable for publication in JSAT and is unlikely to be favorably reviewed by JSAT' reviewers." The National Institute of Drug Abuse responded to my proposal by sending me an application for a grant. I have long been retired. Anyone want to give this grant a try? I even emailed our local investigative reporter suggesting he track down how our millions are being spent on the opioid crisis – no reply. At least I did receive a reply from the Overdose Prevention Coordinator for Florida.

I have a second idea for comparing individual treatments. It involves using both a no treatment group and a placebo against the real treatment. It works as follows:

The Power of Control Groups

The Double Comparison Example

Cognitive Therapy (CT)

Standard is Percent who make 1 year without relapse.

A. No treatment Success rate = 35%

B. Placebo treatment Success rate = 45%

C. CT Success rate = 55%

Therapy is 2.0 times better than placebo.
(55% - 35%)/(45% - 35%)

Motivational Interviewing (MI)

Standard is number of NA meeting over 3 months.

A. No treatment Number of meetings = 3

B. Placebo treatment Number of meetings = 6

C. MI Number of meetings = 12

Motivational Interviewing is 3.0 times better than placebo.
(12-3)/(6-3)

This "Double Comparison" procedure gives you a measure of the strength of the treatment. It even allows two different treatments (standards) to be compared as long as each procedure uses a comparable (greatest) placebo available. Remember, no one study is definitive. If several studies are done, you could determine the average or median strength of the treatment and the range of success. Given limited funds, a placebo that costs one-tenth of a treatment and is 50% as effective might produce better overall results by reaching ten times as many people.

We need a control group for an entire inpatient experience to discover which treatment centers are effective.

Here is a summary of why we cannot rely on evidence-based practices:

Ten Reasons to Distrust Evidence-Based Treatment

1. Many studies do not have a legitimate control group.
2. The evidence might be based on a small number of studies.
3. The evidence may only suggest a small improvement over doing nothing.
4. If only a small percentage of a group make significant gains, the evidence will suggest the treatment works.
5. The treatment being tested may not be well-defined (e.g., family therapy).
6. The evidence may be produced by persons who are more highly trained than the average treatment provider (e.g., college professors who teach the method being investigated).
7. Studies do not always use the same criteria for improvement.
8. Persons who know they are being studied might act differently.
9. What works in the short-run might not work in the long-run.
10. The amount of time given to a treatment procedure might be a big factor in its success.

As of June, 2018, the National Registry of Evidence-Based Programs and Practices has been suspended. However, this suspension is not necessarily related to my above arguments.

What I Recommend for Someone Addicted to Drugs or Alcohol

1. Find yourself an AA or NA sponsor.
2. Get yourself a 24/7 app for help when you need it.
3. Consider using an opioid agonist or antagonist or Antabuse for alcohol.
4. Find yourself a treatment program. I cannot recommend any one in particular because I believe the most important part of treatment is your assigned counselor. The best counselors are not necessarily the most educated or the most experienced. When in doubt, choose outpatient treatment. Note: Private treatment varies from $10,000 to $30,000 per month. One treatment center in my list costs over $1000 per day.
5. Family therapy is important. Let parents, spouse and children give support and talk about how they were affected.
6. If single, find a Sober House to live in after treatment such as Oxford house for recovered addicts. If living elsewhere, attend some type of regular aftercare for a year.
7. Belong to something (church, sports, hobby club, volunteer work).
8. Sometime after at least a year of being sober/clean, <u>get a life</u>! Find things to do that

are meaningful and/or fun. Do not center your life around not getting high.

9. NEVER GIVE UP! Relapses are common. Good things come to those who persist.

What I Recommend for Treatment Centers

1. Have a separate program for readmissions. It is embarrassing for a person to return. Be generous and take the blame. Tell them you have a special program for people who need additional help. I will give you an example of a program for readmissions when I discuss the program I ran.
2. Have at least one home follow-up for those who are no longer coming to weekly group meetings. Home follow-up saves lives. People who do not return for a scheduled follow-up might be dead, in jail or high/drunk. You might catch a person who is close to relapsing or has already done so. Home follow-up allows for continued support and encouragement. Furthermore, seeing a person's home and neighborhood will give you a better idea of what that person is up against. Also, during a home visit you can often get consensual validation from another person who will verify as to whether the client has remained drug free. There is actually something called "Recovery Coaching".

3. Consider also electronic follow-up. In this day and age, 92% of adults have a cell phone and 85% use the Internet. Lauren Stahl, a former addict, created an app called "Sparkite" that helps addiction treatment centers monitor their former clients and lets former clients keep in touch as well as track personal goals. A study done in 2014 found that those with a smart phone app had a recovery rate of 51.9% vs 39.6% for the control group (Gustafson, *JAMA Psychiatry.* 2014;71(5)).
4. Allow clients who are not happy with AA or NA to drop out but not until they find another regular group to attend such as a book club, a bowling league, a bible study group, or a music group, etc. Every group you belong to is a support group!

Addiction is difficult to break on the first try and I believe follow-up is critical. The problem with the medical model is it places most of the resources up front. Let me give you an example. Suppose someone comes to a physician with heart problems. The physician has a lot of great tests to determine the exact nature of the problem. This is followed with the latest medical procedures and/or medication. The patient is then told to change his diet and exercise on a regular basis. A good physician will set up a date in a few months to re-evaluate the patient, especially if he had a $70,000 heart bypass.

Suppose after the one follow-up visit the patient never returns. Instead he sits in front of the television and eats junk food on a regular basis. What happens next? **NOTHING!** I belong to a wellness gym near a hospital. They know exactly how many times a month I exercise from my ID check-in. If I were a heart patient, the gym could send my physician monthly reports of the number of days I exercised each month.

Speaking of gym membership, it has gone up in recent years. If you live in a big city, you probably live within 15 minutes of a gym. Regular exercise will add more years to your life than proper diet. What is the "relapse rate" for gym membership? A 2016 study of 1.5 million YMCA member (MobileFit) discovered that 53.5% terminated their membership in 12 months. If addicts have a relapse rate of over 50% in a year because they are addicts or because they have a chronic illness, what do we call those people who quit the gym? Psychologists (and statisticians) have a name for those people. They are called "normal". One-third of our population is obese. Evidently leading a healthy life is not easy.

I would like to see a study that tried to get those people who left the gym to return – 1/3 by telephone, 1/3 by email and 1/3 by a home visit. I think all of the methods would help but I predict that the home visit would produce more people returning than the first two methods combined.

<u>I believe that most addiction treatment centers need to place more resources on follow-up, even if it means taking away from primary treatment.</u>

What I Recommend the State Governments Do to Fight Addiction

In 2018 the federal government is spending 4.6 billion to fight the opioid crisis. How do I believe the states should spend this money?

1. Create independent diagnostic centers to make treatment recommendations and referrals. By not being in the treatment business, these recommendations would be unbiased. These same diagnostic centers would also be used for mental illness. Many addicts have a co-occurring diagnosis.
2. Do home follow-up of a select sample of persons who were treated for addiction. Every year select a new sample. Again, the state can get honest unbiased relapse rates. In return for treatment center client lists, the state could provide licensure/certification. The state can consistently apply the same standards of improvement for everyone.
3. Provide funds for drugs used in addiction treatment such as methadone, buprenorphine, Naloxone, Naltrexone, Acamprosate, Disulfiram, Bupropion, and Varenicline.
4. Provide funds to addiction treatment centers to provide rewards for contingency management such as clean urine.
5. Provide apps that give 24/7 support, keeps the person in touch with where he received treatment, and/or tracks personal goals set in treatment.

Apps for addiction include Weconnect, Trigrhealth, Sparkite, Quit That, Sober Tool, and Vida.

6. Subsidize post-treatment living facilities for addicts in recovery.
7. Put MBA's in charge of addictions. Physicians and psychologists believe in "evidence-based" practices as found in journal articles and have little interest in saving money.

Florida is receiving 27 million dollars from the federal government. Nowhere in their plan did I find any attempt to gather relapse rates! Same for Louisiana's 24 million dollars (*Times Picayune* 9-26-18).

Recently, I suggested that state licensing boards that certify counselors should require pre and post testing of their clients. In the state of Virginia not a single counselor supported this idea. I spoke before the Texas State Board of Examiners of Psychologists and suggested that they establish a web site for clients to rate their counselors at the completion of therapy. No luck. These professionals do not seem to want to know how effective their work is; at least if it requires effort.

The advantage of the state doing both assessment and follow-up is that they can ultimately see what treatment works for whom. Assessment will include socio-economic status, age of first usage, personality, and peer groups. Follow-up will include a check list of therapies, where received and length of treatment. This is the feed-back needed to improve treatment. Over the years we will know if the treatment for drug addiction is improving.

Women and teenagers are probably the only groups large enough that allow for their own treatment centers. There is some research that indicates that women do better in women-only treatment centers. I recommend women and children needing addiction treatment separate themselves from adult men just to avoid harassment. Both of these groups are subject to victimization. Women on drugs appear to be a cheap source of prostitutes. These women have an increased likelihood of spreading HIV or other sexually transmitted illnesses. They are also more subject to violence. Do countries with legalized prostitution have fewer women on drugs?

Up until the crackdown on opioid prescriptions, the last several years has led to a dramatic increase in opioid abuse among the elderly. Nearly ten times the number of elderlies were prescribed opioids following 1990 than previously. The hospitalization rate for misuse of opioids among the elderly increased more than 150% from 1993 to 2012 according to government reports (https://www.hcup-us.ahrq.gov/reports/statbriefs/sb177). I am not aware of any addiction treatment centers that cater to the elderly. An elderly person is more likely to have cognitive deficits. Surely, a 60-year-old man does not want to be in treatment with people half his age. How much do they have in common?

The state doing referrals should encourage treatment specialists similar to medicine. Private treatment centers currently claim they can treat everyone who has any type of drug addiction. A private addiction treatment center that only dealt with sensation seekers but not trauma victims could not stay in business. With the state making referrals, programs that specialize such as dealing with only women, the elderly, or with a nutrition program or even an arts program, might have a chance of surviving.

What I Recommend the Federal Government Does to Fight Addiction

1. The federal government needs to fund new treatment approaches such as those I have previously mentioned. We should not be satisfied with 40% to 60% drug relapse rates.
2. They should also fund studies to be done by unbiased people to replicate studies that have shown highly favorable results.
3. The federal government should only give money to states who will assess relapse rates for addiction treatment. They should encourage states to set up a systems approach similar to what I have been advocating.

4. The federal government should try cultural solutions like free heroin clinics and teen nightclubs.
5. The federal government should have a continual ongoing taskforce to rate recreational/street drugs on how harmful/useful they are. Suppose they are given a score from 0 (perfectly safe and useful) to 100 (deadly and of no value). The states can now draw their own line as to which drugs are legal. However, if cigarettes have a higher score than marijuana, they can both be legal, they can both be illegal or marijuana can be legal and cigarettes illegal. States could draw the line where they like but there would be no picking and choosing which drugs people favor. (Note: It would be great if a medical task force could do the same for prescription drugs.)

Summary

1. The answer to the question "Are we making progress in the treatment of alcohol and drug abuse?" is **unknown** and apparently will **remain unknown** until we gather legitimate standardized feedback with valid control groups. Without honest relapse rates we will never have a good handle on what works for whom in treating addictions.
2. State agencies should make diagnoses and referrals and also gather relapse rates for addiction treatment centers with samples.

3. Feedback is the way to improve just about anything. I believe that two counselors from the same treatment center can differ greatly on the success of their clients. Florida and Louisiana are receiving millions for "evidence-based" approaches to treating addiction. Unfortunately, they are not talking about their own evidence.
4. I believe addiction treatment centers need a separate program for readmissions and should place more emphasis on follow-up.
5. Addiction treatment studies are of limited value when they compare treatment with no treatment. Journals on addiction should discourage this practice.
6. I believe that cultural changes, such as providing free heroin in a monitored setting and supporting teen "nightclubs", would produce gains far greater than can be achieved by school prevention programs or addiction treatment.

Brainerd State Hospital in Minnesota in the 1970's

Programs

We had three separate programs for alcohol addiction. We only had a small number of patients with other drug addictions, usually in addition to alcohol addiction.

Our main program was based on Alcoholics Anonymous. In other words, it was a 12-step program plus group meetings and individual counseling. Key steps include admitting you are powerless over alcohol, submitting to a higher power, and making amends to those you have hurt.

A second program was geared toward the hard-core alcoholics. Our other psychologist ran a small intense group using the in-depth methods used by therapists. At the time, Transactional Analysis was popular. One dictionary definition of Transactional Analysis "is a system of popular psychology based on the idea that one's behavior and social relationships reflect an interchange between parental (critical and nurturing), adult (rational), and childlike (intuitive and dependent) aspects of personality established early in life." She never used the words "psychotherapy" as we discovered that alcoholics do not like to think of themselves as mentally ill.

Our third program was one I created called "Time Structuring". This program was geared toward readmissions which made up nearly one-third of our clientele. Any addiction, whether drugs, gambling or sex takes up a good portion of an individual's free time. How is a former alcoholic or addict going to fill this void? AA meetings are not enough.

Our clients in the Time Structuring program chose a minimum of three goals/activities. One of these goals consisted of family and community such as a date night with your spouse, attending sports or school events with your children, belonging to a club or church group, or volunteer work.

A second goal involved health such as jogging, dieting, or annual physician checkups. Abstinence was considered a given for most of our clients.

The third goal was one of personal interest. Group members were to choose something they found enjoyable and/or meaningful. These goals were often hobbies such as gardening, reading, playing the piano, etc.

Our Time Structuring program had two Volunteers in Service to America (VISTA). These people visited former clients in their homes to see if they were following up on the goals they set in treatment.

"SAMHSA has delineated four major dimensions that support a life in recovery:

- **Health**— ... healthy choices that support physical and emotional well-being
- **Home**—having a stable and safe place to live
- **Purpose**—conducting meaningful daily activities, such as a job, school volunteerism, family caretaking, or creative endeavors, and the independence, income, and resources to participate in society

- **Community**—having relationships and social networks that provide support, friendship, love, and hope" (www.samhas.gov/recovery).

Our Time Structuring Program at Brainerd State Hospital specifically worked on similar goals. Of course, our program preceded SAMSHA's four dimensions.

Although it would be easy to assume that addicts lack a sufficient number of healthy activities; being an empiricist, I created my own measure. The "Things I Have Done Inventory" contains 132 items in 10 categories plus one Lie scale. The ten categories were Cultural, Service/Political, Social, Outdoors, Sports, Sensual, Hobbies, Building/Repairing, Travel, and Literary/Academic. People who took this inventory responded as to whether they have ever done this activity and if they have done it in the past year. The items were primarily common activities such as "I have subscribed to a magazine", "I have taken pictures with a camera", and "I have performed in a choir, band, or play." This inventory was used by several Minnesota State Hospitals.

The total scores on this inventory were compared between the Mentally Ill, the Chemically Dependent and psychiatric staff. Even when only comparing those with only a high school education, the psychiatric staff (mostly aids) engaged in 27% more activities than the chemically dependent, and 67% more activities within the last year. Complete results of this study are presented in Appendix 8. The importance of healthy activities for addicts appears to be very important. A study on 156 addicts at a methadone clinic reported in *Scientific Mind* (Dec 2007/Jan 2008) concluded that the addicts "level of boredom was the only reliable indicator of whether they would stay clean".

Role Playing

The Time Structuring program had little in common with most treatment approaches to alcoholism. We replaced "talk about your problems" with role playing. It was my experience that many alcoholics are good talkers. They know what to say in treatment, especially readmissions. However, I discovered that many of these good talkers failed at handling everyday situations such as applying for a job, meeting a new neighbor, or having an argument with a spouse.

Of course, we always role played being offered a drink. Several of our patients thought they should tell people up front that they are recovering alcoholics. I thought different. If during role playing a client told a new neighbor he was a recovering alcoholic, I volunteered to play his role. I would introduce myself as a recovering sex addict. I would then add, "I noticed you have an attractive wife." My feeling was that people who know you well will eventually find out that you are a recovering alcoholic. For everyone else, a firm "no thank you" is a sufficient answer when being offered alcohol.

With role playing, the client can play his or her spouse or even a counselor. I enjoyed switching roles. Now the alcoholic had to tell me what would work for him or her. Furthermore, with role playing, any member of the group can suggest a better way to handle a situation. I learned a lot from what others said.

The Time Structuring program differed from the AA program in that we used weekend passes to try out new behaviors, not as a reward for good behavior. It is all too easy to get comfortable in a highly controlled environment.

Social Skills

I believed that social skills training was an underutilized method of treating alcoholics as well as the mentally ill. I taught active listening, conflict resolution, interpersonal skills, visualization for achieving goals, creative problem solving and relaxation techniques. I called my class “Mind Skills”. I had a few patients rank my class as more helpful than medications or counseling. I later adapted these classes for business seminars and the general public via a department store (Joske’s of Texas).

One of the most unusual skills I taught at Brainerd State Hospital was “how to walk”. I would take depressed persons who walked with their heads down and body in tight and teach them to walk proudly with big steps, swinging arms and a smile. Just as your emotions affect your body language, your body language affects your emotions.

We had a psychiatric technician have an afternoon “tea” to teach the mentally ill appropriate social behavior.

Exposure and Response Prevention

Brainerd State Hospital is in northern Minnesota – far outside the Bible belt. Telling our small-town clients to avoid situations with alcohol was unrealistic. So, we ran an experimental group that did the opposite. With a counselor and a Volunteer in Service to America (VISTA), **we took a small group of clients to a bar in the evening!** There they learned to drink nonalcoholic drinks, socialize, dance and play pool. Essentially, we were using the standard therapeutic techniques of desensitization plus exposure and response prevention. Desensitization helps people without alcohol in a bar become comfortable without a fear of being ridiculed. Exposure and response prevention technique helps people lose their craving for alcohol by being exposed to alcohol without drinking. (You could use virtual reality for drug users.) We had one of our clients say he was out on the dance floor while the regulars were drinking to get the courage to ask a woman to dance. I am not aware of any other program that takes alcoholic clients into a bar. Unfortunately, our sample was not large enough for me to submit a journal article before I left Minnesota for a warmer climate.

Bergen, Norway uses a 4-day therapy for Obsessive-Compulsive Disorder (OCD). Two of those days involve prolonged exposure and response prevention. According to the OCD Newsletter, Winter 2018, "More than 90% of the patients have reliably improved while 68% have remitted at 12-month follow-up." "Researchers found that prolonged exposure therapy led to lasting changes in participants' brains that were associated with improvement in PSTD symptoms. About four weeks after therapy ended, fMRI showed elevated activity in the front-most region of the frontal lobe, an area called the frontopolar cortex (*Stanford Medicine News Center*, July 17, 2017).

The success rate of the Time Structuring Program was about the same as our AA program – around 40%. (These numbers are estimated because I do not trust the high figures given by significant others.) Note, the Time Structuring Program was made up mostly of readmissions. We also had more Native Americans in our program. Consequently, we allowed the goal of moderation. If ever a problem called for a cultural solution, it is alcoholism on Indian reservations. Insisting on total abstinence can be setting up some people for failure. I would guess that many people have never even considered the possibility that treatment could make someone worse. Harm reduction is sometimes a better solution than abstinence. Harm reduction is more than moderation; it is keeping someone from driving when high or drunk. It is keeping someone from sharing needles. It is keeping someone sober/clean while on the job.

Brainerd State Hospital's Time Structuring program received an award from the National Institute of Drug Abuse (Appendix 9). All of this was taking place when Hazelden was using confrontation and had no clue as to their success rate.

I regret leaving Brainerd State Hospital before collecting substantial data on the Time Structuring program. I thought that I could run a similar program in

Texas. As it turned out, I could not get a job as a psychologist in Texas. My career as a psychologist lasted less than seven years. My best explanation for this is given in my book *Merit – The Forgotten Dimension in Choosing an Occupation* (Amazon). One of the reasons I came out of retirement to write this book is because I am not convinced that today's treatment programs for the addictions are any better than what we did at Brainerd State Hospital over 40 years ago.

Epilogue

I guess the truth is out. I haven't worked in the field of addiction in 40 years. Even back then, my specialty was alcoholism. Am I arrogant or just crazy to think I can write a book on the opioid crisis? First, it upsets me that politicians who cannot agree on anything have no problem in giving the states money in the hope that the states knew what they were doing.

Second, it infuriates me that it is fine to disbelieve in evolution and global warming when there are hundreds of studies to support these concepts but we can accept that addiction treatment centers in the business of making money are faithfully following the scientific literature.

Third, I think the scientific literature is only a start. I believe the states need to set up their own systems of evaluation and use that feedback to make improvements. Back in 2006 it was written "Better still is a system that monitors the ongoing outcome of services, providing timely, accurate, and reliable feedback to treatment providers, managers, and funding sources as well as to affected individuals and their families" (*Rethinking Substance Abuse*, p. 310). If you agree with me, please email your state official in charge of substance abuse (See Appendix 10). Government, in general, is not known for planning for the future. Politicians want to get credit for immediate gains.

Fourth, we need to create models that simulate communities and models that simulate people. Science is measured by the ability to make accurate predictions.

Showing that method 'A' is statistically significantly better than method 'B' or better than chance is just the beginning. Statisticians do not have true knowledge. They can only tell you what presently works and can predict the future based on the past. Einstein had true knowledge. He predicted that planets bend light before anyone had made that observation. People with true knowledge about substance abuse need to create models that can make predictions that do not rely solely on the past.

To me, giving the states money to lower the number of opioid deaths is comparable to giving the Catholic Church money to prevent sexual abuse by priests. I have already stated why I believe it is a given that opioid deaths will greatly decline in the near future. I also believe that the sexual abuse by priests was solved by Gay Pride. Young homosexuals no longer need to become priests to "cure" their homosexuality and keep others from asking why they are not interested in women. This is another example of the power of cultural change. Nevertheless, I recently read that the Catholic Church has already taken credit for the decline in sexual abuse by priests in the last sixteen years by procedures they implemented in 2002. After receiving a lot of the taxpayers' money, I expect the states will take credit for fewer opioid related deaths.

Medication-Assisted treatment is the "latest" trend in treating opioid addiction. Most professions have a bias. Physicians like medications, counselors like talking cures, social workers like support groups, educators like new ideas to be taught and the clergy prefer a change of heart. Unfortunately, there is not a profession based on teaching skills to those in treatment for addiction or mental illness. Research is great for giving us ideas for treatment, even if new ideas benefit from an enhanced placebo effect. Consequently, program evaluation is necessary to see if the average treatment center for addiction can put the latest trend into action to produce long-term results in the everyday world. Only time will tell.

I thought Antabuse was a good idea in the 1970's. Alcoholics Anonymous, a group that did no research, thought differently. Still, I was able to develop a program that not only had nothing to do with AA but actually allowed moderation as a goal (primarily for young people and Native Americans). Oddly enough, I did not see myself as a trailblazer, just someone following common sense and always searching for the data to back me up. Furthermore, because I had set up a system of program evaluation, I was fully capable of throwing out my own baby if it did not work.

On the other hand, I was naïve enough to think I should be completely honest when applying for a job. More recently, I wrote a book on how to make counseling better and cheaper (*Counseling: A Profession or a Trade?*). No publisher was interested. Although this current book has suggestions for people with addiction problems, these people are not my primary audience. The grass roots are not likely to rise up and demand accountability. Neither is my intended audience the scientific community that relies on grant money for research. My only hope is that someone in a position of authority will take notice. There are fifty states and I would be thrilled if just one of those states decided they needed a true system of referral and follow-up for drug addiction.

What makes this book different from most other books on addiction is that I have no cure for addiction and my suggestions are not going to solve anything in the immediate future. No one at the state level is going to receive any credit for implementing a system of referral and follow-up while gradually getting out of the business of treatment. Can my ideas compete with the promises of the pharmaceutical industry? Can my ideas compete with the many free recovery groups available? Can my ideas compete with the many books that say they have a cure for addiction? Presently, addiction treatment centers and free help groups share the following characteristics:

1) No one will ever know how truly effective they are.
2) No one will ever be able to effectively match a person with the methods most likely to help.

Any way you look at it, addicts choose short-term rewards over long-term gains. How can you expect our federal government to solve our addiction problem when they do the very same thing? Our national debt is over 22 trillion dollars. Two-thirds of our population have not saved enough money for retirement. One-third of our population is obese. Over half of those who join a gym go for less than a year. Choosing short-term rewards over long-term gains is the norm, not the exception.

Government needs to be the first to change. (See Appendix 11).

Most books on addiction are written by physicians, psychologists, and former addicts. They typically base their conclusions on personal experiences, theory, and research involving less than one-thousand persons. Most are overly optimistic. Some even promise a cure. An exception is Judith Grisel, a neuroscientist who wrote *"Never Enough"* (2019, p. 206) who says "I'm not especially hopeful about the prospects of solving something as complex and intractable as addiction anytime soon."

Of the several books I have read on addiction, none explained how it was possible to have non-directive counseling in the 1940's and methadone maintenance in the 1970's and yet we waited forty years before we decided these were good treatments. Without a state system of feedback in place like the one I am recommending; we could be waiting another 40 years to recognize the value of something that exists today. We need a system that would require random samples with valid control groups and in-home follow-up.

In the future with a system of independent diagnosis and referral, treatment, and follow-up; computer programmers and statisticians will do data mining on over hundreds of thousands of cases. They might even find individual differences. With my limited knowledge of addiction, I am sure I said a lot of wrong things in this book. **Measuring what works in the real world is not one of them.**

Appendix 1

The Following tables are from 1975 (put in Excel).

Types of Alcoholics and the Learning Chain

		Type of Alcoholic	Motive	Situation	Response	Consequences - Initial and (Delayed)
1.		Emotionally Immature	Produce a good feeling	Swayed by others	Peer choice	Good feelings
						(Irresponsible actions/impulsive)
2.		Neurotics				
	A.	Anxious	Nervous & tense	Stressful	Quick & reliable relaxer	Relaxation
						(chronic tension/chronic drinking,
						does not face problems
	B.	Depressed	Depression	Failure, loss, rejection	Trouble drowner	Numbness & self-pity
						(Guilt & remorse)
	C.	Character	Need for power, love	Exaggerates need	Easy way to feel a sense of	Decreased inhibition, brings out feelings
			or importance		accomplishment	(short-term effects)
3.		Psychotic	End confusion	Stressful	Available sedator	Numbness & oblivion
						(lowered efficiency)
4.		Cultural	Conformity	Usual pastime	Few alternatives	Sociability
						(progressive efficiency loss and
						related behavior problems)
5.		Way of Life	Most needs	Script	Identification or development	Satisfies many motives
					over the years	(Eventual dissatisfaction of others)

Types of Alcoholics and Treatment Emphasis

Type of Alcoholic	Goals	Primary Means	Secondary Means
Emotionally Immature	Develop Control, forsight and Reason	12 Step Work A.A. club Sponsor Half Way House	Counseling with significant others Industrial assignment Antabuse
Anxious	Learn a new response to anxiety	Relaxation, Meditation Recreation, O.T. Physical Education	Tranquilizer Find a low stress setting
Situational Reaction	Support a person through a crisis	Individual Counseling Community Assistance	Family Counseling
Depressed	Overcome resentments Express feelings	Group Therapy Psyhodrama	Individual Counseling Confrontation Medications
Character-Neurotic	Undecover underlying feelings and needs	Confrontation Character Analysis Relive painful events (Abreaction)	Family Therapy Psychodrama
Cultural	Learn new pastimes Alter environment	Encourage positive interests: hobbies, church, community Education Find a new setting - job, friends Promote community plannning	Teach controlled drinking Treat as immature
Way of Life	Break up game Change script	Family Therapy Eliminate personal rewards related to drinking Encourage new interests	Treat as a character-neurotic
Chronic	Placement in an environment which maximizes existing potential	Develop special well-structured communities for this population	Placement in nursing homes board and care, or family setting

Appendix 2

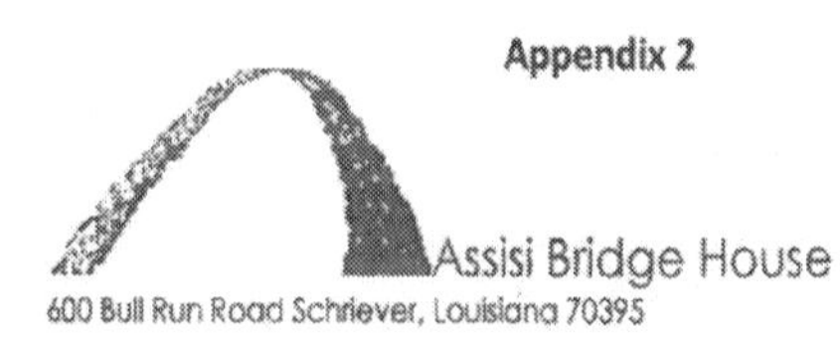

600 Bull Run Road Schriever, Louisiana 70395

Assisi Bridge House

2016 Annual Report

(Admissions from 2015)

Admissions in 2015:	**51 residents**
Rate of Occupancy:	**87% of capacity**
Average Length of Stay:	**101 days**
Length of stay 0 - 30 days:	**9 residents** (18% of the ABH population)
Length of stay 30 - 90 days:	**13 residents** (25% of the ABH population)
Length of stay 90+ days:	**29 residents** (57% of the ABH population)
Sober one year (qualified):	**64%** (16 of 25 former residents with 90+ days who we have been able to contact)
Sober one year (unqualified):	**35%** (18 of 51 former residents. There may be more sober former residents but we have been unable to contact them).

We have been able to stay in touch with 25 of the 29 residents who remained in the Assisi Bridge House for over 90 days. Forty-two percent (64%) of those residents stayed sober for at least one continuous year. The 18 residents reported here sober for one continuous year, represent 35% of the total 2015 admissions of residents. There may be more former residents with one year's sobriety, but we have been unable to contact them.

Independent Living Program

Admissions in 2015:	**7 residents**
Rate of Occupancy:	**52% of capacity (based on 4 beds in a three bedroom apartment)**
Average Length of Stay:	**72 days**
Sober one year (qualified):	50% (2 of 4 former residents with 90+ days who we have been able to contact)
Sober one year (unqualified):	33% (2 of 7 former residents)

2 of the 7 men admitted to the ILP in 2015 stayed sober for one continuous year.

Appendix 3

Addiction Treatment Follow-Up Example

Write-In or Circle Answer/Number

Demographic Data

1. Follow-Up Date: Yr _____ Mn____ Dy___ (1) 6 Mn or (2) 1 Yr
2. Name ___________________ Age ___ Sex: (1) M or (2) F
3. Years of Education ___
4. Family Income: (1) Under $20,000 (2) to $40,000 (3) to $80,000 (4) Over $80,000
5. Marital Status (1) Single/Divorced (2) Married (3) Room Mate
6. Employment: (1) Full-Time (2) Part-Time (3) Unemployed
7. Significant-Other Present at Interview: (1) No (2) Yes
8. If yes, Relationship: (1) Spouse (2) Relative (3) Other

Treatment Data

9. Treatment Facility (see codes) _____
10. Treatment Type: (1) Inpt (2) Outpt (3) Both
11. Goal: (1) Abstinence (2) Harm Reduction (3) Other ____
12. Length of Inpatient Treatment (Weeks): ____ (99) Ongoing
13. Length of Outpatient Treatment (Weeks) ____ (99) Ongoing
14. Individual Counseling Per Week: (1) None (2) Less than one
15. (3) 1 or 2 (4) 3 or more
16. Name of Counselor if known: ______________________
17. Group Therapy Per Week: (1) None (2) Less than one (3) 1 or 2 (4) 3+
18. Was client's family consulted? (1) No (2) Once (3) 2+ (4) Not Applicable
19. Family Therapy Per Week: (1) None (2) Less than one (3) More than one
20. Psychological Testing: (99) None (1) Addiction (2) Personality (3) Both
21. Other Psychological Tests:

    ____

22. Were you treated for a co-occurring disorder? (Check primary one if several) (1) None (2) Anxiety/PTSD (3) Depression (4) ADHD/Learning Disorder (5) Schizophrenia (6) Bi-Polar Disorder (7) Other ______________________________
23. Other Medical Conditions: (1) No (2) Yes

    ____
24. Medication-Assisted Treatment: (1) No (2) Yes
25. If Yes, Medication Used (Add up numbers circled below): (99) Do not know (1) Buprenorphine (2) Naloxone [Suboxone:1+2=3] (4) Methadone (8) Naltrexone (16) Other ______________________
26. How many weeks on above medication: _____ Still taking (99)
27. Attendance in treatment of: (1) NA (2) AA (3) Both (4) Neither (99)
28. If Yes, Per Week: (1) Less than once (2) About once (3) About twice (4) More
29. Check all of the activities you participated in: (Add up numbers circled) ___ (1) Meditation/Mindfulness (2) Music or Art (4) Nutrition Counseling (8) Fitness/Exercise (16) Yoga/Tai Chi (32) Role Playing/Psychodrama (64) Relapse Prevention
30. Check all of the skill training you received (Add up numbers circled): ____ (1) Anger Management (2) Assertive Training (4) Communication Skills (8) Relaxation Methods (16) Interpersonal Skills
31. Additional Therapies/Activities:

    ____

Current Status Since Treatment or Last Follow-Up

32. Use of abused substance(s): (1) None (2) One relapse (3) More than one relapse (4) Presently using
33. Are you still involved with some type of professional treatment?
    (1) No
    (2) Yes ____
34. <u>Monthly</u> attendance of NA/AA: (1) Not at all (2) Once or twice (3) weekly (4) More than once per week
35. If in NA/AA, do you have a sponsor? (1) Yes (2) No
36. If in NA/AA, are you a sponsor? (1) Yes (2) No
37. Religious Attendance: (1) None (2) Sometimes (3) Often (4) Regular

38. Do you follow good nutrition (minimal fast foods, sugars, sodas, fried foods, red meats)? (1) Faithfully (2) Often (3) Sometimes (4) Rarely
39. Do you get plenty of exercise? (1) Faithfully (2) Often (3) Sometimes (4) Rarely
40. How many regular groups do you attend (business, hobby, sports, arts, political, religious such as study groups)? (1) None (2) One (3) 2 or 3 (4) 4 or more
41. How often have you attended sporting events in the last six months? (1) Often (2) Sometimes (3) Rarely (4) Never
42. How often have you attended art events (music, drama, etc.) in the last six months? (1) Often (2) Sometimes (3) Rarely (4) Never
43. Which activities were you a part of in the last six months? (Add up numbers) ____ (1) Outdoors (fishing, hiking, etc.) (2) Playing a sport (4) Working on a hobby (8) Performing (band, theater, etc.) (16) Community service (volunteer)
44. Daily quality time with spouse or partner: (1) Faithfully (2) Often (3) Sometimes (4) Rarely (5) No spouse or partner (6) Don't Know
45. Daily quality time with children living at home: (1) Faithfully (2) Often (3) Sometimes (4) Rarely (5) No children at home (6) Don't Know
46. Conditions of living surroundings: (1) Spotless (2) Neat & Orderly (3) Average (4) Dirty or disorganized (5) A total mess
47. In the interviewer's opinion, close friends and family are (1) Very supportive (2) Somewhat supportive (3) Not supportive (4) Don't know (5) Not applicable

Appendix 4

The following statistics are from "Alternative Hospital Indices" (Robert Kratz and Sidney Nystrom, Hastings State Hospital) and are based on fiscal year 1971-1972. The first numbers are for Brainerd State Hospital. The ranges are given in the parentheses for the eight Minnesota State Hospital programs.

		Mental Illness	Alcohol & Drug
1.	Average length of stay	98 days (98-447)	43 days (34-54)
2.	Length of stay considering readmissions	151 days (151-632)	67 days (53-94)
3.	Cost per day	$19.06 ($15.54-24.54)	$17.11 ($14.67-21.61)
4.	Average cost per hospitalization	$1868 ($1868-$8913)	$736 ($649-$963)
5.	Workload index	5.4 (3.2-5.4)	12.1 (9.0-19.8)
6.	Net Patient turnover index	67 (34-67)	85 (52-85)
7.	% of patients discharged who stay out of the hospital	46% (42%-59%)	45% (27%-50%)
8.	"Cure" index	1.71 (.48-1.71)	3.82 (1.81-4.82)

2. Formula: (length of stay) * (1 + readmission rate)

5. Formula: $\frac{\text{\# annual admits + \# patients}}{\text{\# staff}}$

6. Formula: $\frac{\text{(\# discharged - \# readmissions)}}{\text{(\# new admits + \# initial patients)}}$ * 100

7. Formula: $\frac{\text{(\# of discharged - \# readmissions)}}{\text{(\# discharged)}}$ * 100%

8. Formula : $\frac{\text{(\#discharges- \#readmissions)}}{\text{(average \# of patients)}}$

Appendix 5

Counselor Evaluation by the Client

(An Example: To be done anonymously on-line)

Name of your Counselor: ____________________

Today's Date: M __ D __ Y __

Approximate number of weeks you were in counseling:

_____

Your Sex: M __ F __ Your Age Range: Below 20 __ 20-29 __ 30-39 __ 40-59 __ Over 60 __

First Time in Counseling? Y __ N __

Answer the following questions according to this guide:

1 = Never, 2 = Seldom, 3 = Sometimes, 4 = Often, 5 = Always

1. Did your counselor make you feel comfortable? __
2. Was your counselor a good listener? __
3. Was your counselor judgmental? __
4. Did your counselor give advice? __
5. Did your counselor assign homework? __
6. Did your counselor help you set goals? __
7. Did your counselor explain his or her approach to counseling? Y __ N __
8. Did your counselor ask to speak with someone who knows you? Y __ N __
9. Did your counselor work with you on developing exit criteria (i.e., what needs to happen that will make you ready for discharge?) Y __ N __
10. Did your counselor do any testing? Y __ N__

11. Did your counselor or you chart any specific behaviors? Y __ N __
12. Did your counselor refer you to any other source of assistance? Y __ N __

Answer the following questions according to this guide:

1 = not at all, 2 = very little, 3 = somewhat, 4 = very much, 5 = extremely

13. How knowledgeable would you rate your counselor? __
14. How helpful would you rate your counselor? __

Comments:

____

____

____

Appendix 6

The Times-Picayune

ASHTON PHELPS
Chairman of the Board 1967-1983

Issued every Sunday by The Times-Picayune Publishing Corp. at 3800 Howard Ave., New Orleans, La. 70140

YOUR OPINIONS | Letters

Making sure the 'War on Drugs' is successful

Kenner

All this talk about the "War on Drugs" sounds reminiscent of the Great Society of the 1960s, when people were willing to spend money on social reform without any solid evidence to indicate that these efforts could be successful.

Right now the bulk of the anti-drug money goes to law enforcement, which is primarily geared toward stopping the supplier. Two rather dubious assumptions underlie this emphasis.

The first is that when one supplier is caught, another supplier will not simply take his place. Because enormous sums of money are involved with drug trafficking, going after suppliers is an endless task.

The other is that reducing the supply of drugs will reduce the consumption of drugs. There may be some truth in this assumption, but it seems likely that the first people to cut back their drug use when supplies are limited are not the people who create the most problems to our society. Ironically, the short supply of drugs could in theory lead to more break-ins and robberies to pay for their increased cost.

Of the $13.6 billion already allocated to fighting drug abuse, about 23 percent went for treatment and prevention. President Bush's proposal would up this to about 30 percent.

Shifting the emphasis from law enforcement to treatment will be a better idea when we have more confidence in the effectiveness of our treatment programs. Having directed a program for alcohol and drug rehabilitation, I can affirm that treatment programs are certainly better than doing nothing although remission rates are very discouraging.

Drug education is another target for federal money. Most schools already have drug education programs. The effect education can be expected to have on drug abuse depends on the extent to which drug abuse is a result of ignorance. We know the impact of sex education on stopping the growing number of teen-age pregnancies has been minimal. We cannot expect drug education to fare much better.

If law enforcement, individual treatment and comprehensive education are not likely to yield a high return on the dollar what is left? Use of propaganda is another strategy for reducing drug usage.

Although propaganda is a negative word for many people, it needs to be distinguished from education. Education is presenting people with facts so that they can make their own decisions. Propaganda works by giving people the motivation to make a choice in a certain direction.

There can be a fine line between education and propaganda, as evidenced in anti-smoking literature. Nevertheless, "Just Say No To Drugs" clearly falls under the category of propaganda. It is precisely our recent experiences with national anti-smoking efforts that demonstrate the potentially high return rate of a massive propaganda campaign.

What has our campaign to reduce smoking taught us? First, the baseline research on treatment programs for smokers indicated that giving up smoking was no easier than giving up alcohol. Second, the initial results based on surveys made it appear that anti-smoking efforts were of no value. Some point of critical mass must be reached before positive results occur. When that point is reached, momentum builds followed by a gradual leveling off.

From 1976 to 1989, the percentage of people who smoke dropped over one-third. The prominence President Bush and others have given to the war on drugs puts us in a position to maximize the propaganda effect.

President Bush has called cocaine use our most serious problem. A possible innovation for dealing with cocaine use is for undercover law enforcement officers to infiltrate areas of known users and distribute previously confiscated cocaine mixed with ingredients to make the user temporarily nauseous.

The use of aversive conditioning for drug abuse is not new. Its effects could have a lot more impact when done surreptitiously. This strategy can be launched simultaneously with a "No High To Buy" propaganda campaign.

Jay Alexander

Appendix 7

Standard Addiction Treatment

1. Psychiatric Services: Detoxification, Medication Assisted Treatment, Medications for co-occurring disorders
2. Psychological Services: Counseling (Individual, Group and Family), Motivational Interviewing, Role Playing, Abreaction, Behavioral (Contingency Management, Goal Setting, Exposure and Response Prevention, Systematic Desensitization, Aversive Conditioning)
3. Skill Training: Conflict Management, Anger Management, Assertive Training, Communication, Interpersonal, Relaxation, Mindfulness, Meditation
4. Education: Drug education, Lectures, School attendance, Reading
5. Health: Nutrition, Exercise, Yoga, Tai Chi, Supplements
6. Vocational: Job Training, Finding employment, Industrial assignments
7. Support Groups: AA/NA and other addiction support groups, Religious attendance, Service groups, Special Interests groups
8. Cultural: Music, Art, Dance, etc.
9. Recreation: Sports, Hobbies and various activities
10. Follow-Up: Relapse prevention, Drug testing, Electronic connections (apps), Sober house
11. Miscellaneous: Providing transportation, Babysitting, Legal assistance

Appendix 8

Things I Have Done Inventory

Objective: Determine the disparity in the breadth of leisure time activities among the mentally ill, the chemically dependent, and others (psychiatric staff). _Methods:_ A 132 item "Things I Have Done" inventory of leisure activities was administered to the mentally ill, chemically dependent, and psychiatric staff at a state psychiatric hospital. _Results:_ Even controlling for education, the psychiatric staff had been engaged in 25 percent or more activities than the patients and nearly twice as many in the past year as measured by this inventory of common activities. Small positive correlations were found between activity totals and education (r=.41) and activity totals and income (r=.39). No significant differences were found in total activity scores between the mentally ill and the chemically dependent; or between males and females; or between the young and the old; or between married or unmarried. *Conclusions:* It is suggested that a simple measure such as the 132 item "Things I Have Done Inventory" would be helpful for testing whether assisting and encouraging psychiatric and chemically dependent patients to develop leisure time activities will improve post-hospitalization adjustment and reduce readmissions.

Things I Have Done – Study Results

TOTAL SAMPLE

Table 1 – Anytime

	N	Type	Avg	Stnd Dev	Groups	T-Test
Mentally Ill	55	M	69.0	23.8	M/C	0.5157
Chemically Dependent	56	C	71.9	23.5	C/S	0.0000
Psychiatric Staff	37	S	103.2	17.0	M/S	0.0000
	148					

Table 1 – Last Year

	N	Type	Avg	Stnd Dev	Groups	T-Test
Mentally Ill	47	M	26.5	20.5	M/C	0.7305
Chemically Dependent	44	C	27.9	18.1	C/S	0.0000
Psychiatric Staff	37	S	50.7	18.5	M/S	0.0000
	128					

HIGH SCHOOL EDUCATION

Table 1 – Anytime

	N	Type	Avg	Stnd Dev	Groups	T-Test
Mentally Ill	22	M	69.8	21.1	M/C	0.1646
Chemically Dependent	22	C	79.5	24.0	C/S	0.0015
Psychiatric Staff	9	S	101.3	10.7	M/S	0.0000
	53					

Table 1 – Last Year

	N	Type	Avg	Stnd Dev	Groups	T-Test
Mentally Ill	21	M	24.8	16.1	M/C	0.5909
Chemically Dependent	19	C	28.0	21.0	C/S	0.0147
Psychiatric Staff	9	S	46.7	15.3	M/S	0.0028
	49					

Appendix 9

Award from the National Institute of Drug Abuse

1975

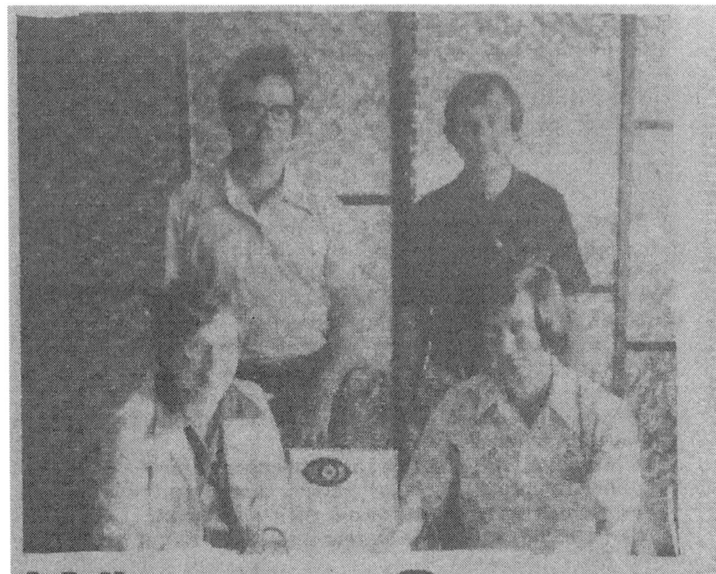

Wierman Gets Hospital Award

Dr. John Wieriman, -psychologist at Brainerd State Hospital received an award from the National Search Panel of the National Institute of Drug Abuse on June 25th. A year long effort was made to find drug prevention programs that have an impact on youth. Dr. Wieriman is advisor for the Time Structuring Program. Offered as an alternative to the traditional treatment program for the chemically dependent, this method assists persons to find and maintain constructive and interesting activities to replace the time formerly spent in drinking and taking drugs. This project will be featured in the National Directory of Youth Alternatives to Drug Abuse. Guidelines used by the Panel in their selection of programs were: innovativeness, replicability and degree of youth involvement.

Appendix 10

Substance Abuse Agencies

State	Email
AL	Diane.Baugher@mh.alabama.gov
AK	randall.burns@alaska.gov
AZ	tom.betlach@azahcccs.gov
AR	charlie.green@dhs.arkansas.gov
CA	jennifer.kent@dhcs.ca.gov
CO	nancy.vandemark@state.co.us
CT	Miriam.Delphin-Rittmon@ct.gov
DE	elizabeth.romero@state.de.us
DC	doh@dc.gov
FL	Ute.Gazioch@myflfamilies.com
GA	cassandra.price@dbhdd.ga.gov
HI	edward.mersereau@doh.hawaii.gov
ID	anduezar@dhw.idaho.gov
IL	Maria.Bruni@illinois.gov
IN	kevin.moore@fssa.in.gov
IA	kathy.stone@idph.iowa.gov
KS	Sharon.Kearse@ks.gov
KY	Michele.Blevins@ky.gov
LA	james.hussey@la.gov
ME	sheldon.wheeler@maine.gov
MD	Barbara.Bazron@maryland.gov
MA	Allison.Bauer@state.ma.us
MI	Renwickt@michigan.gov
MN	brian.zirbes@state.mn.us
MS	melody.winston@dmh.state.ms.us
MO	mark.stringer@dmh.mo.gov
MT	bperkins@mt.gov
NE	sheri.dawson@nebraska.gov

NV	jpeek@health.nv.gov
NH	Joseph.P.Harding@dhhs.state.nh.us
NJ	valerie.mielke@dhs.state.nj.us
NM	wayne.lindstrom@state.nm.us
NY	certification@oasas.ny.gov
NC	flo.stein@dhhs.nc.gov
ND	psagness@nd.gov
OH	tracy.plouck@mha.ohio.gov
OK	tlwhite@odmhsas.org
OR	royce.a.bowlin@dhsoha.state.or.us
PA	emhostette@pa.gov
RI	rebecca.boss@bhddh.ri.gov
SC	sgoldsby@daodas.sc.gov
SD	Tiffany.Wolfgang@state.sd.us
TN	marie.williams@tn.gov
TX	rachel.ashworth-mazerolle@dshs.texas.gov
UT	dothomas@utah.gov
VT	cynthia.thomas@vermont.gov
VA	jack.barber@dbhds.virginia.gov
WA	imhofC@dshs.wa.gov
WV	Elliott.H.Birckhead@wv.gov
WI	Joyce.Allen@wisconsin.gov
WY	chris.newman@wyo.gov
Potus	https://www.whitehouse.gov/contact/
GOV	mariel.lifshitz@samhsa.hhs.gov
Data	daryl.kade@samhsa.hhs.gov

Appendix 11

Cooking Lobsters

Why Things Get Worse Before They Get Better

J. Alexander Wieriman

We have all heard that by raising the temperature little by little, a lobster becomes a meal without realizing what is happening. My premise is that the most serious issues we have to face are those that creep up on us and we do not act until they become crises. Some of these issues include:

Federal Deficit
Personal Debt
Immigration
Collapse of Infrastructure
Obesity
Divorce
Crime
War
Global Warming/Oceans rising
Pollution
Poor Health

Axiom 1: We are genetically programmed to respond to immediate threats to our survival.

Corollary 1: People who solve problems get a lot more recognition than people who prevent them.

Rescuing a drowning person from a flood makes you a hero. Saving a thousand people from flooding by effective flood control gets you no recognition at all. People who handle crises rise up in the ranks. Being the mayor of New York during the September 11th crisis places you in contention to run for a higher office. Twelve U.S. presidents were generals. People remember war-time presidents. What would be the status of Abraham Lincoln if it were not for the Civil War? FDR is well known because of the Great Depression. Eisenhower became president as the result of being a general during World War II. As a president he was often referred to as the "do nothing" president. However, during his administration he created the interstate highway system that probably created more wealth than any other president. This wealth was generated long after he was in office when trucking took over the railroads as the chief means of product distribution. I would like to say that Eisenhower showed great foresight. Actually, he created the national highway system under the concept of defense. By law, most of the interstate system must be straight so that an airplane can land on it.

Rule 1 (The Cardinal Rule): It is better to prevent a crisis than to solve one.

This rule requires little explanation. Crises are costly. If you wait until that mole on your back become skin cancer you will have wished you had it removed earlier. An ounce of prevention is worth a pound of cure. When you look at a crisis in terms of dollars, this aphorism is an understatement. For example, by not following its own safety rules, British Petroleum had to spend over a billion dollars correcting an oil spill in the Gulf of Mexico. By not keeping down the federal deficit, we now pay millions in interest.

Axiom 2: Men fight wild beasts and each other; women raise children, gather food and prepare meals. In other words, men are programmed to respond to immediate danger while women need to prepare for the future.

Corollary 2: Men (or women like men) should carry out and enforce the plans that women (or men like women) make.

Prediction 1: The first woman president of the United States will have all of the characteristics of a man. In other words, she will not be the type of leader we need.

Rule 2: Unless there is a crisis, put a planner in charge.

Most captains of industry are still men and the United States is one of the few industrialized nations to have never had a woman in charge as president. We elect generals (12) and lawyers (25) to our highest office. These are people who see the world in an adversarial way. Voters like strong take-charge leaders. Women are more likely to rule by consensus. It may take longer to reach decisions by consensus but implementing them becomes easier.

Axiom 3: Maturity is the ability to delay immediate gratification for greater long-term gains.

Corollary 2: Leaders take credit for short-term gains and blame the previous leader for long-term problems.

Most CEO's are interested in making gains while they are still in charge. Stockholders want to see results quarterly. Consequently, most people do not consider maturity to be a desirable trait for a leader. We want what we want and we want it now!

I remember when young people lived in an apartment before they bought their "starter home". At that time the average home was about 1400 square feet. Now it is about 2400 square feet. The housing collapse of 2009 was fueled by people who over-bought with the encouragement of realtors and bankers.

Axiom 4: Consensus through diversity is an effective way to come up with the best solution to a problem.

Many studies have demonstrated that the decisions of a group exceed the decisions of any one individual for complex problems. Manager training seminars often ask people to choose what they need to survive in a hostile climate such as the desert or the arctic. When the group works together to reach a consensus to a problem, they invariably do better than the solutions of individuals.

Corollary 4: Diversity as practiced by most businesses is not diversity at all.

If you want to create a diverse group, you need to first decide on what dimensions the group should differ on and then measure people. A group consisting of individuals of different sex, color, or national origin guarantees nothing! If you are not sure how to measure diversity for selection to a committee, I would suggest you have the candidates each take the Myers-Briggs Type Indicator test. This test classifies people into one of 16 personality types. The test rates people on the four dimensions of introversion-extraversion, sensation-intuition, thinking-feeling, and perceiving-judging. To ensure a diversity of opinion, make sure that each person on the committee has a different personality type.

Axiom 5: The smaller the organization, the more efficient it is.

We all know about the problems with large bureaucracies. Too many levels of management with upper management too far removed from the day to day operations. Furthermore, bureaucracies have lots of committees that produce too many rules and regulations. Recently, the countries of the world were rated as to the best places to live based on health, education, and business climate. The top-rated countries were all small!

Corollary 5: It is the nature of organizations to continually expand until they fall by their own weight.

Wal-Mart has destroyed small town businesses that cannot compete with the large discounts they get as the result of their size. **The fact that Wal-Mart can sell goods for less because of these discounts does not make them efficient.** Many a company has gotten rich from gobbling up smaller companies. The reason small companies exist at all is because they are usually more efficient and quicker to take action. Innovation can occur rapidly in a small company. General Motors was not the first to produce efficient cars when they were in demand or SUV's when the public wanted those. Fewer layers of bureaucracy and personal service will always allow small companies to compete.

Axiom 6: We take action when a problem reaches the breaking point.

Some breaking points are clear cut. When a bridge collapses, we realize we need to put more effort in inspecting our bridges and making repairs. Having a number of bridges on the verge of collapse doesn't do the trick. No one gets credit for preventing a crisis. When people die, we take notice. Most breaking points are vague. How many illegal immigrants do we need to have before this problem becomes a priority?

Corollary 6: We will always need problem solvers in charge if we never have planners to keep crises from happening in the first place.

Solutions to cooking lobsters

Action Points:

The simplest way to avoid the tremendous loss from creeping problems is to define an "action point". For example, suppose you are a person who constantly worries about your weight. The way to reduce your worries is to decide to take action if ever your weight exceeds a certain number. Once a month you should weigh yourself and if you are below the action point you forget about your weight until the next month. There is a method called Statistical Process Control (SPC) that can help you decide when a system is "out of control". SPC is one of the reasons for the tremendous strides the Japanese made in quality control after World War II. Quality control helped Toyota surpass GM in the number of automobiles sold in the world.

Our government should have action points. For example, taxes should automatically go up when X number of troops are deployed outside of the United States. This way we would pay as we go for military action instead of building up a huge debt. Some actions, such as retiree pay, are already tied to the Consumer Price Index. Minimum wages should also be tied to the Consumer Price Index. It would probably be a good idea if the treasury rate went up or down by a formula. That way a committee would meet only in cases when this formula needs to be over-ruled.

Proportional Response:

Proportional response requires a response in proportion to change that has taken place. For example, a weight gain of ten percent might require a ten percent reduction in your daily calorie intake. One of the problems with governing by catastrophe is that a catastrophe calls for drastic measures and drastic measures lead to public revolt.

Planned Replacement:

When I was young, someone told me to pay for my first automobile with cash. Then I should put a little money aside each month for my next car. That way I would never have to finance an automobile. When I worked in data processing for the United States government, we paid for our data processing equipment with "Planned Replacement" funds. Whenever the government builds a bridge, they need to set aside a small amount of money for replacing or repairing that bridge.

Savings:

Clearly one of the best ways to save money is to avoid interest charges as pointed out above. Whenever someone asks me if I am for a balanced budget I always reply "no". After a few awkward stares I then explain that I am not for a balanced budget because I believe the government should take in more than it spends. I would still be living in a trailer if I spent every penny I ever made. As a nation the United States is not a believer in savings. Furthermore, our parents probably saved a greater proportion of their income than we do. Savings is nothing new. Moses had the Egyptians store grain for the bad years.

Rule 3: Create Long Term Goals:

Presidents are not believers in long term goals because they want to get credit for their actions while in office. The same goes for company CEO's. The way to get around this is for unelected committees to meet and work out long-term goals. Term limits is another solution. Supreme Court justices have the options to go against public opinion. Public opinion will never favor long term goals. Too many people live from pay check to pay check. They do not want to put money aside for infrastructure, upgrading technology, and that proverbial rainy day.

Fortunately, every individual can put something aside, even if it is only pocket change. Putting a small amount aside that earns interest is invaluable, especially when you start this habit with your first job. So what if your friends think you are poor when you do not buy that house and car you can barely afford. It is only a matter of time before you pass them up.

Rule 4: Invest in Knowledge and Skills

Everyone needs basic skills in communication and problem solving. Some things are learned by having a formal education. Most skills, however, are passed down to you from someone else. Early generations put more of an emphasis on being a jack of all trades. They saved a lot of money by not hiring repairmen. Certain skills, such as cooking and carpentry, will always have value in the best and worst of times. How many older people have said they had wished they had learned to play piano when they were young?

Axiom 7: No one knows the value of a college education.

The only way to assess the value of a college education would be to randomly pick some people to go to college while others are randomly excluded from college. Without random assignments, studies that show college graduates make more money are meaningless. These studies do not even control for intelligence and social class.

Rule 5: Pick a Mate Who Shares your Long-Term Goals

A grasshopper and an ant make a poor combination. Two ants do not go together any better when one ant loves the city and the other the country. Sharing values is important but it is not the same as sharing long term goals.

People without long term goals choose the best paying job and the best-looking mate offered now. Choose the job, the location, and your partner that is the most compatible with where you want to be down the road and be patient.

Axiom 8: Follow your Dream but be Prepared First

Prediction 2: The National Debt will eventually create a financial catastrophe causing one of the largest Stock Market drops in history.

So, What's for Dinner?

Appendix 12

Placement of References in a Book

I place my references within the text because I find it exasperating to be constantly thumbing to the back of the book. I look for two things in a reference. First, I look at the source. If the source is a newspaper or popular magazine, I have a low confidence in what is said. If the source typically summarizes an area of research such as Psychological Bulletin or Scientific American, I have a high confidence in what is said. If the source is a specialized journal, I have a medium confidence is what is said.

Second, I look at the date of publication. People who do research are usually aware of earlier studies in their subject matter. Consequently, I place a higher confidence in studies that are the most recent.

Because my references are within the text, I usually give only enough information to find the original article. This would be the principle author's name, title and date for a book. For a journal article I would give the principle author's name, the year, volume and issue numbers. Journal articles often have long titles so I would give them only if I thought they added valuable information. References to internet addresses are tricky as some can be exceedingly long.

I cannot find any research on the percent of people who read the references when they are at the end of a book or on the percent of people who will actually look up an original article referenced. Do publishers even verify that the author accurately reflects the references? Although I have nothing against the standard APA format for references, I have no idea as to why a publisher would insist on this.

Made in the USA
Columbia, SC
20 May 2025